OVERCOMING AND HEALING CANCER

Inspiring True Stories of Recovery

Chunmei Yao

happylife GmbH

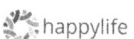

Copyright © 2024 Chunmei Yao

Responsible for the content

happylife GmbH
Dorfstrasse 7A
9495 Triesen
Liechtenstein

Email address: info@happylife.li
Company website: https://happylife.li
LI commercial register: FL-0002.704.829-6
VAT number: 62917
Authorized representative: Chunmei Yao

Image Sources

The images used in this work are licensed through Canva, with some created using DALL-E. All images are subject to applicable terms of use and may not be reproduced, resold, or otherwise utilized without prior permission.

Disclaimer

The information, text, graphics, images, and other materials provided in this book are for reference purposes only and do not constitute medical advice, diagnosis, or treatment. Furthermore, they are not intended to establish a doctor-patient relationship. Under no circumstances should the content of this book be used as a basis for self-diagnosis, medical advice, consultation, treatment guidelines, or a substitute for professional medical care. The author and all contributors to this book maintain a neutral stance regarding the content and viewpoints expressed herein. Individuals utilizing the information in this book are responsible for their own interpretation and application of such information. We explicitly disclaim any liability for losses, damages, injuries, or claims arising from the use of the information contained in this book. The content of this book is based on the successful experiences of individuals who combined scientific discoveries with various therapeutic approaches during their journey of advanced cancer treatment. It is intended to provide reference and inspiration. Due to individual differences, the outcomes described in this book may not apply to everyone and should not be construed as universally applicable medical advice or guarantees. For any health concerns or before taking any medical actions, you are strongly advised to consult a qualified healthcare professional. This book explicitly does not provide an alternative to conventional medical treatment or professional medical advice.

Plagiarism Check

November 12, 2024

We hereby declare that Overcoming and Healing Cancer: Inspiring True Stories of Recovery, published by Chunmei Yao, has undergone thorough plagiarism checks to the best of our ability. Based on our current knowledge and judgment, we confirm that this work is 100% free from plagiarism. We have made every effort to ensure the originality of its content.

CONTENTS

Title Page

Copyright

Preface

Chapter 1: Understanding Cancer – Causes and Risk Factors — 2

Chapter 2: Confronting Cancer – Diagnosis and Emotional Response — 15

Chapter 3: Seeking Scientific Approaches to Confront Cancer – Wise Decisions and Choices — 28

Chapter 4: The Journey of Conquering Cancer – A Guide to Self-Reconstruction — 40

Chapter 5: Unlocking the Body's Healing Potential – Wisdom and Practice — 49

Chapter 6: The Power of the Mind – Emotional Support and a Victorious Mentality — 152

Chapter 7: The Path to Recovery – Real Stories and Reflections — 168

Chapter 8: Renewal and Transformation – Rebuilding Health and Life — 180

Chapter 9: Unwavering Belief – Hope for Recovery and a Vision for the Future — 196

Chapter 10: The Gift of Hope and Wisdom – Reflections and Shared Insights — 224

Chapter 11 : Academic Resources and References – Scientific Knowledge and Support for Health — 266

Afterword	280
About The Author	282
Acknowledgments and Gratitude	286

PREFACE

Welcome to Overcoming and Healing Cancer: Inspiring True Stories of Recovery.

This book captures the remarkable journey undertaken by two cancer warriors. In the face of an unrelenting diagnosis, life's countdown had begun—not only a grim declaration of the illness's toll but a heavy blow to their desire to survive. Under the weight of multiple diagnoses, they rose from the depths of shock and despair, choosing to stand resilient. With unwavering determination and steadfast belief, they have written an inspiring and deeply moving legend of resilience.

Readers witness how the human spirit finds a glimmer of light even in the darkest moments, embarking on a path to a brighter future. Their moving experiences form more than just personal chapters of their lives; they serve as a beacon for all—an enduring message that even in the bleakest of times, hope can be ignited to light the way forward.

Explanation of Pseudonyms

To safeguard the privacy of the individuals featured in this book and to make the content more universal and relatable, we have chosen to use the pseudonyms "Leo Martin" and "Julia Meyer." These names represent their courageous journeys in confronting illness, imbuing their stories with broader resonance and a deeper capacity for empathy.

The Motivation Behind This Book

We are fully aware that when life is at its most harrowing, every struggle is profoundly etched with pain. Yet, it is in these dark moments that individuals often tap into a profound inner resilience and gain the resolve to move forward. Spiritual resilience becomes a vital source of strength in this process. The heroes of this book demonstrate that even from the deepest valleys, one can rekindle the flame within and walk a long, challenging road with unshakeable resolve. We believe these stories will not only bring warmth to your journey but also inspire wisdom and courage, helping you renew your fortitude during challenging times.

Who This Book is For

Centered on Leo and Julia's process of rebirth, this book aims to offer multiple perspectives and practical insights to those facing a fierce battle with cancer and to their supporters, helping them cultivate confidence and handle various challenges with composure. Whether you are currently fighting against illness, seeking ways to improve health and quality of living, or simply looking to read an inspiring, thought-provoking true story, this book offers invaluable insights, practical guidance, steadfast support, and a steady source of motivation. It is not only a steady wellspring of support and inspiration but also a carefully crafted, practical guide for navigating health challenges and pursuing lasting well-being.

Leo Martin's Key Insights

Through experience, we have come to understand the critical importance of taking timely and suitable actions, particularly for those facing advanced stages of illness. This is a race against time, and finding effective methods while acting swiftly can positively impact the overall outlook. To facilitate quick access to key insights, Chapter 5 compiles the personal practices and mind-body management strategies that guided us towards recovery —all of which are backed by scientific research and rigorous validation. The remaining chapters also offer insights from Eastern and Western medical wisdom, the latest advancements in cancer treatment, and expert advice from renowned medical professionals, professors, and leading public health institutions across multiple countries. Each chapter comes together to provide a broad spectrum of encouragement and healing pathways, offering deep and comprehensive support for your journey of renewal.

Why This Book Matters

We believe that this book goes beyond information—it is a guide for lasting positive change, helping you find new strength and resilience amidst adversity. Through detailed accounts of a process from despair to restored health, it shows how to kindle inner strength in life's darkest moments and discover fresh directions in seemingly impossible situations. This is not only a personal story of recovery but a tribute to the resilient human spirit.

Conclusion

We sincerely hope this book can serve as a guiding light on your journey to overcome cancer. Our experiences have shown that, no matter how harsh fate may seem, faith and determination can lead us to renewal. If you are currently battling cancer or supporting a loved one along this difficult road, please remember—you are not alone.

No matter how overwhelming the challenge, we firmly believe that faith and courage will guide us toward a brighter future. May this book offer you, or anyone enduring a difficult time, warm encouragement, unwavering support, and the opportunity to reclaim your strength, imparting the wisdom and confidence to progress toward health. Because every moment is worth treasuring, and each rekindled resolve is a beacon lighting our way.

Together, let us stand strong and welcome every miracle life has to offer.

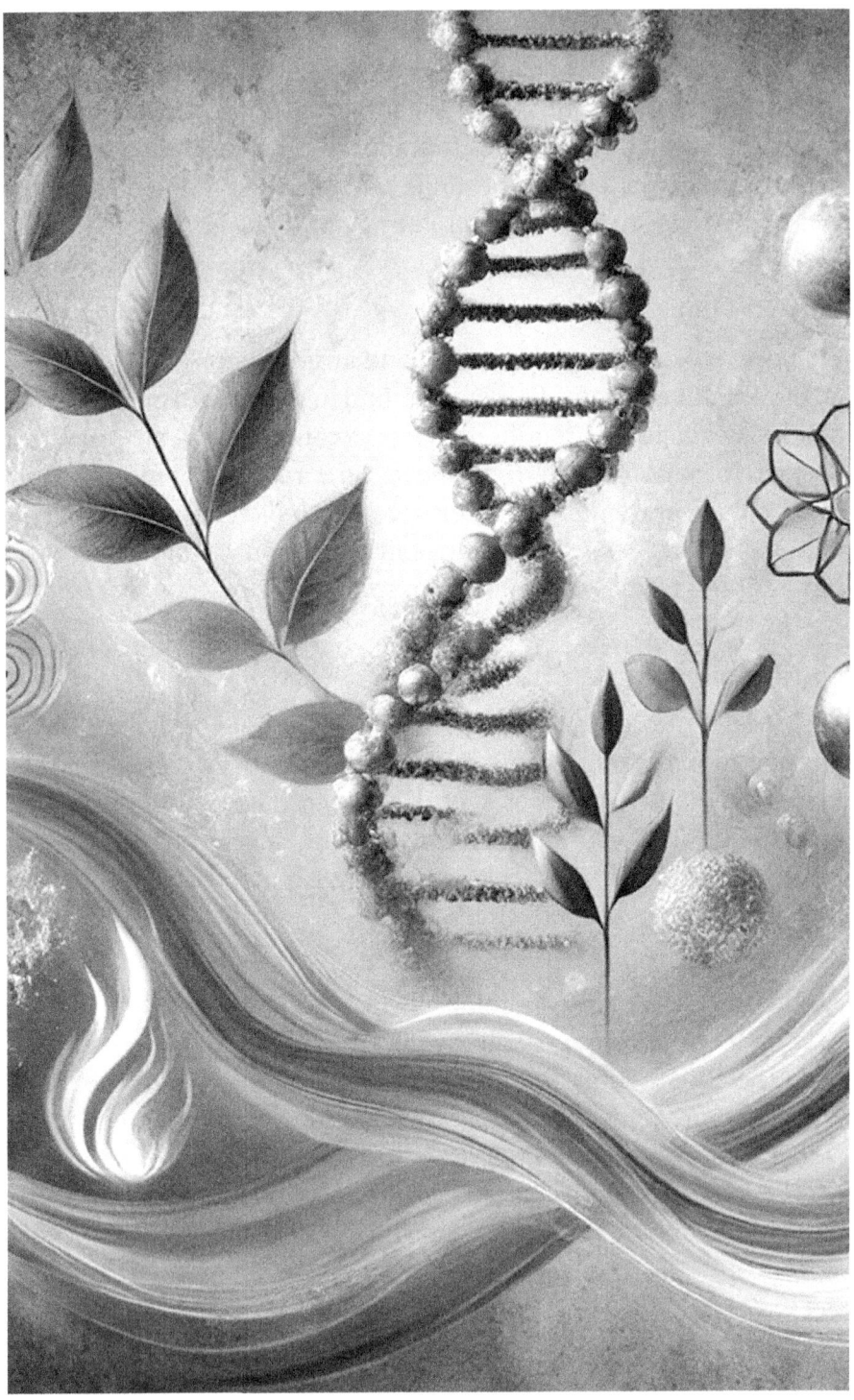

CHAPTER 1: UNDERSTANDING CANCER – CAUSES AND RISK FACTORS

A study published in The British Medical Journal Oncology in 2023 indicates a growing trend of cancer affecting younger populations. The data show that over the past 30 years, the number of newly diagnosed cancer cases among individuals under 50 worldwide has increased by 79%, while cancer-related mortality in this group has risen by 27.7%.

According to the Global Cancer Statistics released in April 2024, nearly 20 million new cancer cases were recorded globally in 2022, with approximately 9.7 million cancer-related deaths. These alarming figures underscore the vast impact and severe threat that cancer poses as a major public health challenge.

Cancer resembles a silent war, relentlessly and rapidly deteriorating human health. These statistics not only highlight the high incidence of cancer but also call for greater emphasis on prevention and effective response strategies.

Notably, the American Cancer Society reports that the incidence of certain cancers, particularly pancreatic, kidney, and small intestine cancers, is rising significantly among younger populations. This trend presents serious new challenges for global healthcare systems, while also driving heightened public awareness about cancer prevention and overall health management.

For many families, cancer represents not only a test of physical health but also an immense financial and psychological burden. When confronted with the challenges of cancer, individuals and their families often face difficult decisions: whether to continue treatments that may cause pain and hardship or to forgo them in favor of spending their remaining time at home with dignity. These decisions are complex, involving professional medical judgments, personal beliefs, and deep emotional considerations. Each family must weigh these factors carefully to make the choice that best aligns with their values and circumstances.

While cancer is often associated with mortality, we must recognize that it is not always an irreversible condition. In fact, many do not pass away due to the spread of cancer cells but because of misunderstandings about the illness or prematurely abandoning treatment. Maintaining a positive outlook, receiving comprehensive support, and having access to accurate information are key to overcoming cancer.

In reality, numerous stories of individuals overcoming cancer—including the experiences of "Leo Martin" and "Julia Meyer" shared in this book—demonstrate that no matter how daunting the challenge, hope should never be abandoned. Every moment of perseverance has the potential to bring a turning point and renewed light.

Therefore, the following content will explain cancer from both traditional Chinese medicine (TCM) and Western medicine perspectives, offering readers a deeper understanding of the disease.

Traditional Chinese and Western medicine each offer unique insights and approaches in addressing cancer. Western medicine, grounded in modern science, targets cancer cells directly through surgery, radiation, and chemotherapy to swiftly inhibit their growth. Traditional Chinese medicine, on the other hand, emphasizes a holistic approach, viewing the causes of disease as closely linked to internal imbalances and focusing on strengthening the body's self-healing abilities to restore health fundamentally. By approaching cancer from these distinct perspectives, TCM and Western medicine provide a more comprehensive understanding of the disease. Integrating the strengths of both can lead to a more profound and informed approach to managing cancer.

Traditional Chinese Medicine's Perspective on Cancer and Its Causes

In the TCM framework, there is no direct term for "cancer." Instead, the disease is described through concepts like "Qi stagnation" and "blood stasis" that depict pathological states within the body. To explain cancer's origin from a TCM perspective, the progression might be summarized as follows: Deficiency → Cold → Dampness → Congealing → Stasis → Blockage → Tumor → Cancer.

In essence, cancer can be seen as the cumulative result of "stasis" and "blockages" within the body, which form the foundation of TCM diagnostics and treatment. TCM therefore views cancer not as a single disease but as a manifestation of an overall imbalance in the body. Health, from this perspective, depends on the balance of Yin and Yang, the harmony of Qi and blood, and the interactions among the Five Elements (metal, wood, water, fire, and earth).

TCM's understanding of illness is deeply rooted in thousands of years of Chinese cultural and medical theory, perceiving disease as a result of both internal and external factors disrupting the body's equilibrium. When external pathogens (such as dampness, heat, cold, dryness, and wind) invade and disturb this balance, disease may arise. For instance, excessive dampness within the body can lead to fluid retention, causing "phlegm-dampness" and impairing spleen function, thereby resulting in various illnesses. Therefore, TCM considers dampness as "the root of all illnesses."

Next, we will further explore the potential causes of cancer from the perspective of Traditional Chinese Medicine (TCM):

1. Yin-Yang Imbalance

Yin and Yang represent two interdependent yet opposing forces that govern everything in the universe, including physiological functions within the human body. According to TCM, maintaining a balance between Yin and Yang is essential for sustaining health. An imbalance can disrupt bodily functions, leading to various health issues, including cancer. When Yin and Yang fall out of harmony, the immune system may be weakened, increasing vulnerability to disease.

2. Qi Stagnation

In TCM, "Qi" (Qì) symbolizes the body's vital energy and plays a crucial role in supporting various physiological functions. "Stagnation" refers to the obstruction of Qi flow within the body. TCM holds that the smooth movement of Qi is vital for health; when Qi becomes stagnant, it can lead to poor circulation of blood and bodily fluids.

3. Blood Stasis

Blood stasis refers to the impaired circulation of blood, causing it to accumulate and stagnate in certain areas of the body, hindering its natural flow. TCM views prolonged blood stasis as a potential cause of hardened masses or lumps, which may develop into more serious health concerns, including cancer. Blood stasis is considered a root cause of many diseases and is particularly associated with tumor formation.

4. Weakness of the Zang-Fu Organs

The term "Zang-Fu" in TCM encompasses the body's internal organs, including the spleen, liver, kidneys, heart, and lungs. When Zang-Fu organ functions are weakened, the body's defense mechanisms may decline, increasing the risk of cancer. For example, spleen deficiency can lead to fluid retention, potentially creating conditions that contribute to tumor formation.

In traditional TCM theory, the human body, mind, and environment are regarded as an interconnected whole, with cancer seen as the result of multiple contributing factors. Additionally, TCM emphasizes the close relationship between emotions and physical health, recognizing emotional imbalance as a key factor in disrupting bodily harmony and triggering disease.

One of the most important classics of Chinese medicine, the Huangdi Neijing (The Yellow Emperor's Inner Canon), written over 2,000 years ago, states: "Joy injures the heart, anger injures the liver, fear injures the kidneys, worry injures the spleen, and shock injures the gallbladder." This phrase reflects TCM's deep understanding of the connection between emotions and internal organs. Each emotion is closely linked to a specific organ, suggesting that prolonged negative emotions disrupt the circulation of Qi and blood in the body, weaken immune function, and increase susceptibility to illness. Even "joy," generally considered a positive emotion, is viewed in the Huangdi Neijing as potentially harmful if excessive, as it can disturb the heart's energy, affecting its regular function.

This further illustrates the TCM concept of the "mind-body unity," where mental states directly impact physical health. Thus, maintaining balanced emotions and emotional stability is not only crucial for organ health but also serves as an important method of disease prevention.

In summary, TCM's approach to health focuses on promoting the smooth flow of Qi and blood, maintaining and restoring Yin-Yang balance, and strengthening the Zang-Fu organs to support overall wellness. Additionally, TCM emphasizes addressing underlying causes to prevent the further development and recurrence of cancer.

The Western Medical Perspective on Cancer and Its Causes

In Western medicine, cancer is considered a complex, multifactorial disease involving biological, psychological, and sociological factors. The hallmark of cancer lies in the abnormal proliferation of cells, which can invade nearby tissues and potentially spread to distant organs. Typically, Western medicine views cancer as a disease triggered by genetic mutations; when these mutations cause cells to lose normal growth control, they may proliferate and spread throughout the body.

From a Western medical perspective, the potential causes of cancer include the following:

1. Microbial Infections

Invasion by bacteria, viruses, fungi, or parasites can lead to infections that cause tissue damage and inflammatory responses, ultimately increasing the risk of cancer.

2. Genetic Factors

Gene mutations or abnormalities can disrupt normal biological processes, making the body more susceptible to other carcinogenic factors. Certain genetic mutations can significantly raise the risk of developing cancer.

3. Environmental Factors

Long-term exposure to pollutants, radiation, and other environmental factors can disrupt biological processes, increasing the likelihood of chronic diseases such as cancer.

4. Lifestyle

Unhealthy lifestyle habits can damage cellular structures, causing persistent chronic inflammation, which in turn markedly increases cancer risk.

5. Age

The incidence of cancer increases with age. This phenomenon is closely linked to the accumulation of cellular mutations, the gradual decline of immune function, and reduced efficiency in DNA repair mechanisms. Older cells are more likely to be exposed to various carcinogenic factors over their lifespan, thereby significantly raising the risk of cancer.

6. Immune System

Immune system dysfunction can weaken the body's ability to combat cancerous cells. When the immune system fails to identify or eliminate these abnormal cells, they may continue to proliferate and accumulate genetic mutations, potentially leading to cancer.

7. Psychological Factors

Chronic stress, anxiety, and depression may indirectly increase cancer risk by weakening the immune system. Psychological and physical health are closely connected, with studies showing that a positive mental state can help boost immunity, whereas prolonged psychological stress may heighten the risk of cancer.

In summary, Western medicine generally views cancer as the result of genetic mutations, which can lead to uncontrolled cell proliferation, spread, and ultimately, metastasis. Cancer can occur in any tissue of the body and affects individuals of all ages. Unlike TCM, which attributes cancer to imbalances in Qi and overall energy flow within the body, Western medicine focuses more on the roles of genetic and environmental factors. Despite their differing theories, these two systems can complement each other, offering those affected by cancer a broader range of approaches for management and care.

In the following section, we will explore the differing explanations of tumors within the frameworks of traditional Chinese and Western medicine:

Chinese and Western medical systems each offer unique perspectives on the types and causes of tumors based on their respective theoretical foundations. Western medicine typically explains tumor characteristics and development through pathology and molecular biology, whereas traditional Chinese medicine approaches the causes and symptoms of tumors from a holistic perspective, focusing on imbalances in Qi and blood, as well as dysfunctions of the internal organs.

The Interpretation of Tumors in Traditional Chinese Medicine

From the perspective of Traditional Chinese Medicine (TCM), as previously discussed, the formation of tumors is generally viewed as the result of multiple factors working together, including Qi and blood imbalances, dysfunctions of internal organs, and invasions of external pathogenic influences. Unlike Western medicine, which categorizes tumors as "benign" or "malignant," TCM emphasizes a holistic view and symptom analysis, focusing on bodily balance and the circulation of Qi and blood. Tumors are considered a manifestation of internal imbalance, such as Qi and blood stasis or Yin-Yang disharmony.

In TCM, benign and malignant tumors are primarily understood through diagnostic methods based on "deficiency," "excess," "cold," and "heat":

Benign Tumors

In TCM, benign tumors are generally regarded as accumulations of pathological products such as Qi stagnation, blood stasis, or phlegm-dampness. These tumors typically grow more slowly and have a relatively minor impact on the body. Treatment for benign tumors focuses on regulating Qi and blood, promoting meridian flow, and using methods that remove stasis, regulate Qi, and resolve phlegm, gradually alleviating symptoms and achieving the effect of "softening and dispersing masses."

Malignant Tumors

Malignant tumors in TCM are usually associated with complex patterns of cold and heat, dual deficiencies of Qi and blood, or Yin-Yang imbalances. When treating malignant tumors, TCM emphasizes addressing deeper systemic imbalances with a strategy based on supporting the body's vitality and dispelling pathogenic factors. Treatment is complemented by nourishing Yin, replenishing Qi, strengthening the spleen, and benefiting the kidneys, thus enhancing the body's self-healing capabilities and inhibiting tumor progression.

The Western Medical Interpretation of Tumors

The primary distinctions between benign tumors, malignant tumors, and cancer lie in their growth behavior, development patterns, and impact on the body. These differences are crucial for determining treatment approaches and prognosis.

The explanations are as follows:

Benign Tumors

Growth Behavior

Benign tumors typically grow slowly and remain confined to the tissue where they originated without invasive behavior. They tend to grow locally, are unlikely to become malignant, and rarely spread to other parts of the body. Most benign tumors are encapsulated by a fibrous membrane, which separates them from surrounding tissues.

Growth Type

These tumors grow only within one area and, although they may exert pressure on nearby structures, they pose relatively low risk and usually do not invade or damage surrounding tissues. While benign tumors may persist in the body for many years, in rare cases, they can transform into malignant tumors.

Impact on the Body

Generally, benign tumors pose a minimal threat to health. However, if they press on critical organs or nerves, they may cause discomfort, though they are rarely life-threatening.

Malignant Tumors

Growth Behavior

Malignant tumors grow rapidly and are highly invasive, capable of penetrating and destroying surrounding healthy tissues, posing a significant threat to life.

Growth Type

Malignant tumors are metastatic, meaning they can spread to other parts of the body through the bloodstream or lymphatic system, forming new lesions elsewhere, which makes them particularly destructive.

Impact on the Body

Unlike benign tumors, malignant tumors are life-threatening due to their metastatic and invasive nature. They can impair the function of affected organs, spread to other organs, create new, hard-to-control growths, and make treatment more challenging, often resulting in a poorer prognosis.

Cancer

Cancer is a general term for malignant tumors; however, not all tumors are cancerous. The hallmark characteristics of cancer are rapid growth, invasiveness, and the ability to spread (metastasis).

Cancer not only damages local tissues but also weakens the immune system, causes bleeding, and harms essential organs, ultimately posing a serious threat to life.

Conclusion

This chapter provides an in-depth exploration of the fundamental concepts and causes of cancer from an integrative perspective that combines both Western and Traditional Chinese Medicine (TCM), offering individuals affected by cancer and their families a comprehensive framework for understanding the disease. Western medicine addresses cancer through modern medical technology, focusing on pathological mechanisms, while TCM emphasizes a holistic view and the balance of the body. Understanding the multifactorial causes of cancer is essential for developing appropriate recovery and health support plans. By integrating the strengths of both approaches, those affected by cancer can gain a more complete understanding of their condition, explore suitable response strategies, and improve quality of life and recovery prospects.

For further information on this topic, please refer to Chapter 11, Academic Resources and References: Scientific Knowledge and Support for Health, which includes a variety of resources on cancer and integrated health management from both Western and TCM perspectives. It also contains valuable insights on the treatment approaches utilized by "Leo Martin" and "Julia Meyer" in their cancer journeys. This material serves as a scientifically grounded and effective resource for individuals affected by cancer and for anyone seeking to improve their health.

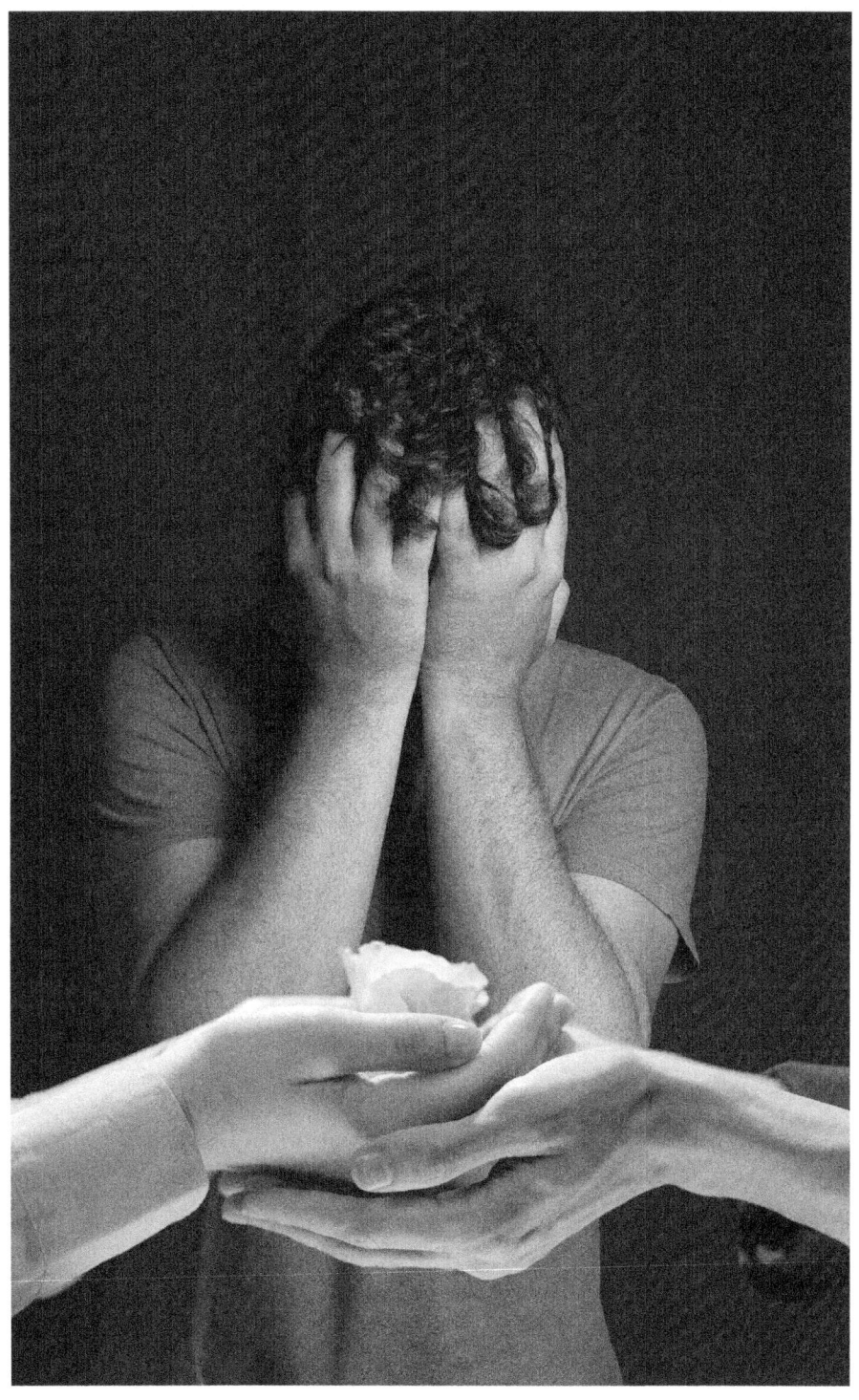

CHAPTER 2: CONFRONTING CANCER – DIAGNOSIS AND EMOTIONAL RESPONSE

When the diagnosis of cancer, especially advanced cancer, strikes like a sudden storm, it inevitably brings a profound psychological shock. Although I cannot fully experience the emotions of those who live through this moment, it is not hard to imagine that it feels like a lightning bolt on a clear day, shattering the calm of their lives in an instant. In that moment, it is as though the whole world falls into darkness, where everything is overshadowed by uncertainty, bringing an overwhelming weight and deep-seated fear.

The emotional impact is so intense that many find themselves plunged into a deep chasm of helplessness and confusion. In mere seconds, plans and visions for the future seem to vanish into an abyss of the unknown, leaving behind an unprecedented void and unease. Even years later, those who have successfully recovered often find it difficult to forget the impact of that moment—a memory etched deeply into their lives, a permanent reminder of life's fragility and unpredictability.

Responses to a cancer diagnosis vary widely, reflecting both an individual's internal journey and the profound choices they make in facing life. Some lose their way instantly, drowning in anxiety and overwhelming pressure, struggling to withstand the abrupt upheaval. They need time to process and come to terms with it, while for others, accepting this reality is a long process, one that might even span a lifetime, leaving them in a prolonged state of disorientation and despair.

However, there are also those who, in the face of cancer, exhibit remarkable resilience and composure. They choose to confront their fear, transforming the intense psychological strain into inner strength, and seeking even the faintest glimmer of light in the darkness. This inner resilience gradually helps them regain control over their lives, allowing them to restore inner balance, sometimes finding a deeper and more fulfilling sense of self than before. It is this strength that sustains them, enabling not only a victory over cancer but also a renewal of life's equilibrium and vitality.

This strength becomes a beacon, guiding them through the darkness and empowering them not only to survive cancer but also to derive new meaning and value from the experience. This profound transformation brings a newfound appreciation for life—each day becomes precious, and every smile and embrace are cherished.

The Inspirational Journey of Mr. Leo Martin: From Cancer Diagnosis to Triumph

Eleven years ago, I was diagnosed with advanced colon cancer—a devastating blow that struck like a sudden storm, shattering the peaceful life I had known. In an instant, everything familiar crumbled, and waves of fear, uncertainty, and despair flooded my heart. Yet, I was fortunate. Today, I am here to tell my story in person: I not only overcame cancer, but I also emerged with a newfound vitality and health that I had never experienced before.

My journey from a diagnosis of late-stage cancer to recovery has been a complete transformation of my life. Along this path, I learned how to persevere through life's storms and to cherish each moment of every day. The fear and helplessness I felt then remain vivid memories. Those days and nights of relentless struggle are deeply etched into my heart, becoming an indelible part of my life.

Standing here today, reflecting on those dark years as I embrace a new lease on life, I feel an overwhelming mixture of emotions: a profound understanding of hardship, as well as the relief and gratitude that come with overcoming illness and embracing renewal. This journey was filled with countless challenges and hardships, but these very trials made me stronger and more resolute.

In Chapter Eight, I will share how I learned to treasure life, finding strength and joy in each present moment. I hope to convey a message through this story: cancer can be beaten, and the hope for recovery is real. Every act of perseverance and each small victory brings you closer to healing. I hope my story inspires everyone who is fighting cancer to believe in themselves and hold onto hope, for each courageous step forward lights the way ahead.

Early Signs and Warning Signals: Recognition and Prevention

It was an ordinary day in May 2013. I went to the hospital for a routine blood test due to a mild viral infection, thinking it was nothing more than a minor episode that would resolve itself in a few days. The doctor prescribed some medication, and I naturally assumed that the symptoms would subside shortly, allowing life and work to continue as usual. However, events unfolded in a way I never expected. During this routine examination, the doctor unexpectedly detected abnormalities in my bloodwork. Out of caution, he recommended a more comprehensive examination at a larger hospital.

Although I felt a vague sense of unease, I quickly reassured myself that it was likely just a random anomaly and nothing serious. Yet, as the results of further tests began to surface, I realized the situation was far more complex than I had imagined. At that moment, a sense of alarm steadily grew within me, like the forewarning of an impending storm.

This unexpected discovery profoundly taught me a vital lesson—health is never something to be taken for granted. Even the slightest physical irregularities can signal potential risks. Looking back at my initial indifference and self-reassurance, I recognize this as a common reaction when people encounter early signs of cancer. In fact, the early symptoms of many cancers are often subtle and easy to overlook, sometimes dismissed as minor issues. Unfortunately, underestimating these warning signals can lead to missed opportunities for timely diagnosis and treatment.

Reflecting on this experience now, I deeply understand that had I not pursued further examinations at the time, the condition might have silently worsened. Therefore, recognizing physical abnormalities early and acting decisively may be the key to preventing and overcoming cancer. Every persistent signal from the body deserves our attention, as it might represent the last line of defense for safeguarding health. This experience not only transformed my attitude toward health but also made me realize that every warning sign from the body is a precious reminder of the value of life.

The Moment of Diagnosis: Facing the First Shock

Following further examinations at the hospital, the doctor delivered news that would upend everything: "You have been diagnosed with advanced-stage colon cancer, and the cancer cells have spread to multiple parts of your body." His tone was somber and grave. Though he refrained from explicitly stating how much time I might have left, the weight of his words made the severity of the situation unmistakable. He strongly urged me to be admitted immediately for urgent medical intervention. As someone who has always prided themselves on staying calm and rational, I instantly grasped the gravity of the diagnosis—this revelation struck like a sledgehammer, shattering the calm rhythm of my life without mercy.

In the moment I heard the diagnosis, my heart sank and then began to race uncontrollably. It felt as though time itself had come to a standstill. Fear surged through me like a tidal wave, sending a deep chill from my core to every part of my body. My stomach churned, my hands trembled involuntarily, and my vision blurred. I struggled to focus on the doctor's every word, trying to process the sudden and harsh reality through logic, yet deep inside, a silent resistance grew. I couldn't accept the cruel blow I had just been dealt. Everything familiar seemed distant and alien, as though the room was spinning and my surroundings had become surreal and detached from reality. This overwhelming numbness engulfed me, leaving me with a profound sense of helplessness, as if I had been thrust into a nightmare I had no control over.

It's impossible to say how long I remained in this daze before I gradually regained some sense of awareness. A flood of uncontainable questions consumed my thoughts: "How could this happen? Why me?" Almost instinctively, I whispered to the doctor, "Are you sure?" He nodded firmly, extinguishing the last flicker of hope I had been clinging to. In that instant, a deafening hum filled my mind, and my thoughts splintered into fragments. I felt utterly lost, unsure of how to face this unforeseen catastrophe.

Despite the deep resistance within me to accept this harsh reality, I clung to a sliver of hope and decided to seek a second opinion at another hospital. However, fate offered no reprieve—the devastating diagnosis was confirmed once again. At that moment, I truly understood how life can be upended in an instant. The overwhelming sense of powerlessness and lack of control made me experience, for the first time, the relentless and unpredictable nature of fate.

Emotional and Psychological Responses to the Diagnosis: Inner Struggles and Adjustment

In the depths of helplessness and fear, I gradually came to realize that only by confronting this illness head-on could I find the strength to keep moving forward. Yet, in the days that followed, I felt engulfed by a dense fog of despair and uncertainty, trapped in a state of profound confusion, almost consumed by the oppressive weight of these emotions. Each day became a battle within, my mind overwhelmed by a flood of thoughts and tormented by endless questions and hypothetical scenarios. Again and again, I asked myself, "What can I rely on amidst all of this?" Thoughts of my aging parents, young child, and cherished friends brought an overwhelming sense of helplessness as the life I once knew seemed to crumble before my eyes.

How could I possibly explain this to them? Unfinished ambitions and unrealized dreams lingered in my mind, refusing to fade. On one hand, I reflected on what meaningful things I could still accomplish in the time I had left; on the other hand, a faint but fierce flame of defiance began to burn within me, unwilling to easily yield to fate. I rejected the finality of the doctor's prognosis and refused to let despair dictate my life.

Following medical advice, I began undergoing routine radiotherapy and chemotherapy. However, two months later, my condition showed no significant improvement. In July 2013, I faced a four-hour surgery, followed by continued radiotherapy and chemotherapy as part of the traditional cancer management protocol. During this arduous journey, I not only attended daily treatments but also remained actively involved in managing my business affairs. I even persisted in pursuing a construction project I had been preparing before my diagnosis—a project that had long been a personal dream.

The groundwork for the project had already been laid, with documents approved and the foundation set. Just as I was ready to commence construction, the cancer diagnosis loomed like an invisible barrier, blocking my path forward. Despite the challenges of post-surgery recovery and the uncertainties ahead, I refused to abandon the project. It became a symbol of my resilience in the face of adversity, an anchor that motivated me to keep going. Immersing myself in the planning and construction process offered a temporary escape from pain and fear, filling me with a renewed sense of purpose.

For me, building this house was not merely about fulfilling a dream; it became a lifeline, sustaining me through my darkest moments. It represented my unwavering determination and hope, serving as a vital source of strength that helped me reclaim my belief in life. This project gave me the courage to face challenges head-on and refuse to bow to fate.

The Journey After Diagnosis: Perseverance and Resilience

From the moment of diagnosis to the initiation of medical interventions and my first surgery, I endured nearly six months of torment. However, my condition not only failed to improve but progressively worsened. Eventually, in November 2013, I had no choice but to undergo a second surgery. Despite immense physical and emotional suffering, I never allowed despair to completely consume me. Perhaps it was the constant demands of my packed schedule that left me little room to dwell on negative emotions. I firmly believed that only by cooperating fully with the doctors could I have a chance of overcoming cancer.

As a senior engineer, I was accustomed to tackling challenges with rational and structured thinking. During my fight against cancer, this logical mindset became an essential pillar of my mental strength. Even during the most painful and chaotic moments, I made every effort to remain calm and take control of the situation. Yet, no matter how resilient one may seem, moments of vulnerability are inevitable. Negative emotions would occasionally surge, leaving me overwhelmed and anxious. But each time, I gritted my teeth and pressed on. I couldn't allow myself to give up—not on myself, not on my family, friends, or everything I cherished. Nor was I willing to bid farewell to this world so easily.

Each follow-up appointment filled me with dread, bringing endless speculation and uncertainty. At times, the process left me feeling lost and disoriented, as though my life had been stripped of its direction. I found myself trapped in a relentless struggle between hope and despair. Each day felt like trudging through an unlit abyss, with no sense of light or bearings. Yet, amidst this darkness, my desire to live grew ever stronger, as if it were the only faint but persistent force propelling me forward.

In January 2014, when I was physically and emotionally exhausted, I faced another devastating blow. During a routine check-up, the doctor informed me that they had done everything they could, but my remaining time was limited. He estimated that I had only six to twelve months left. If I continued chemotherapy, I might extend my life by another six months, though even that came with no guarantees. This news struck me like a final verdict, shattering me completely. I refused to accept such an outcome and began to question the accuracy of the prognosis.

Taking a deep breath, I confronted the doctor with two critical questions: "Can chemotherapy cure cancer? Does chemotherapy cause cancer?" His answers left me both shocked and disheartened. In that moment, I felt as though the entire world had turned against me. It became clear that traditional medicine could no longer provide the solutions I needed. I realized I had to take a different path. With that decision, I resolved to leave the hospital and seek alternative approaches. While I understood the immense risks involved, staying in the hospital felt like a descent into hopelessness and even a potential acceleration of my decline.

I will never forget that afternoon. The doctor warned me that leaving the hospital was extremely dangerous. He said, "If you discharge yourself, you may experience severe pain or post-surgical complications that could force you to return before nightfall." But I had made up my mind. I didn't want to argue further or spend another moment in that hospital. I signed the discharge papers, ready to face a road full of unknowns and challenges. Despite the looming trials ahead, I resolved to bear the consequences of my choice, however daunting they might be. With a faint but unwavering determination, I set out to seek a miracle, prepared to confront whatever lay ahead on this uncharted path.

The Reactions and Support of Family and Friends:

Emotional Anchors

Since my cancer diagnosis, the reactions of my family and friends mirrored my own: shock, disbelief, and at times, an inability to accept the harsh reality. Fear and uncertainty cast a shadow over everyone. Some entered a temporary state of denial, attempting to downplay the severity of the illness and offering me every bit of comfort they could muster. Others firmly held onto the belief that miracles were possible, consistently providing me with hope and encouragement. Like me, they needed time to process, understand, and come to terms with the unexpected blow.

Seeing my loved ones feel powerless in the face of my suffering stirred a complex mix of emotions within me. They did their utmost to soothe my fears, patiently listened to the details of every medical update, and made every effort to stay by my side, offering unwavering emotional support. The time I spent with them became incredibly precious, especially given the uncertainty of how much time I had left. Even though they knew their efforts might not change the course of the illness, they supported me without hesitation. Despite my attempts to appear strong in front of them, the relentless series of setbacks inevitably caused emotional turbulence.

Throughout my battle with cancer, the understanding and support of my family and friends became an indispensable source of strength. Their presence not only brought me inner peace but also significantly alleviated my anxiety and depression, sparing me from feeling isolated or helpless. Their emotional warmth and practical assistance helped me navigate countless challenges in my daily life, proving to be vital throughout the entire journey. Their empathy and unwavering support, in particular, allowed me to maintain a semblance of calm under immense pressure—a mindset that had a profound impact on my recovery.

As time went on, my family remained my strongest pillar of support. With their backing, I discovered the inner resilience needed to confront adversity. They provided me with a constant flow of comfort, encouragement, and warmth, ensuring that even during my darkest moments, I could summon the courage to persevere. It was the love and care from my family and friends that nourished my heart and soul, offering me boundless motivation to keep moving forward with courage and determination.

Conclusion

In this chapter, we explored the profound emotional impact of a cancer diagnosis on individuals and their families. From the recognition of early symptoms to the shock of diagnosis, each step carries an immense psychological burden. A cancer diagnosis not only shatters the world of the person receiving it but also deeply unsettles their family and friends, plunging them into fear and uncertainty.

The early detection of cancer symptoms is crucial, as it provides invaluable time for prompt diagnosis and preparation for the treatment ahead. Equally significant is addressing the psychological impact that follows a diagnosis. Emotional fluctuations and mental strain are inevitable for both the individual and their loved ones. Consequently, adopting proactive strategies for psychological adjustment and emotional resilience is essential to navigating this journey more effectively.

We emphasized the pivotal role of family and friends in coping with cancer. Their companionship, support, and encouragement not only serve as a powerful emotional anchor but also play an indispensable role in the process of managing the illness and pursuing recovery. While family members cannot bear the physical suffering of their loved one, their support often stabilizes emotions, alleviates anxiety and loneliness, and provides the strength and motivation to endure even the toughest moments.

Through this discussion, we have gained a deeper appreciation for the value of emotional support and a strong social network. These factors not only empower individuals facing cancer to find the strength to continue their fight but also rekindle their hope and confidence in life.

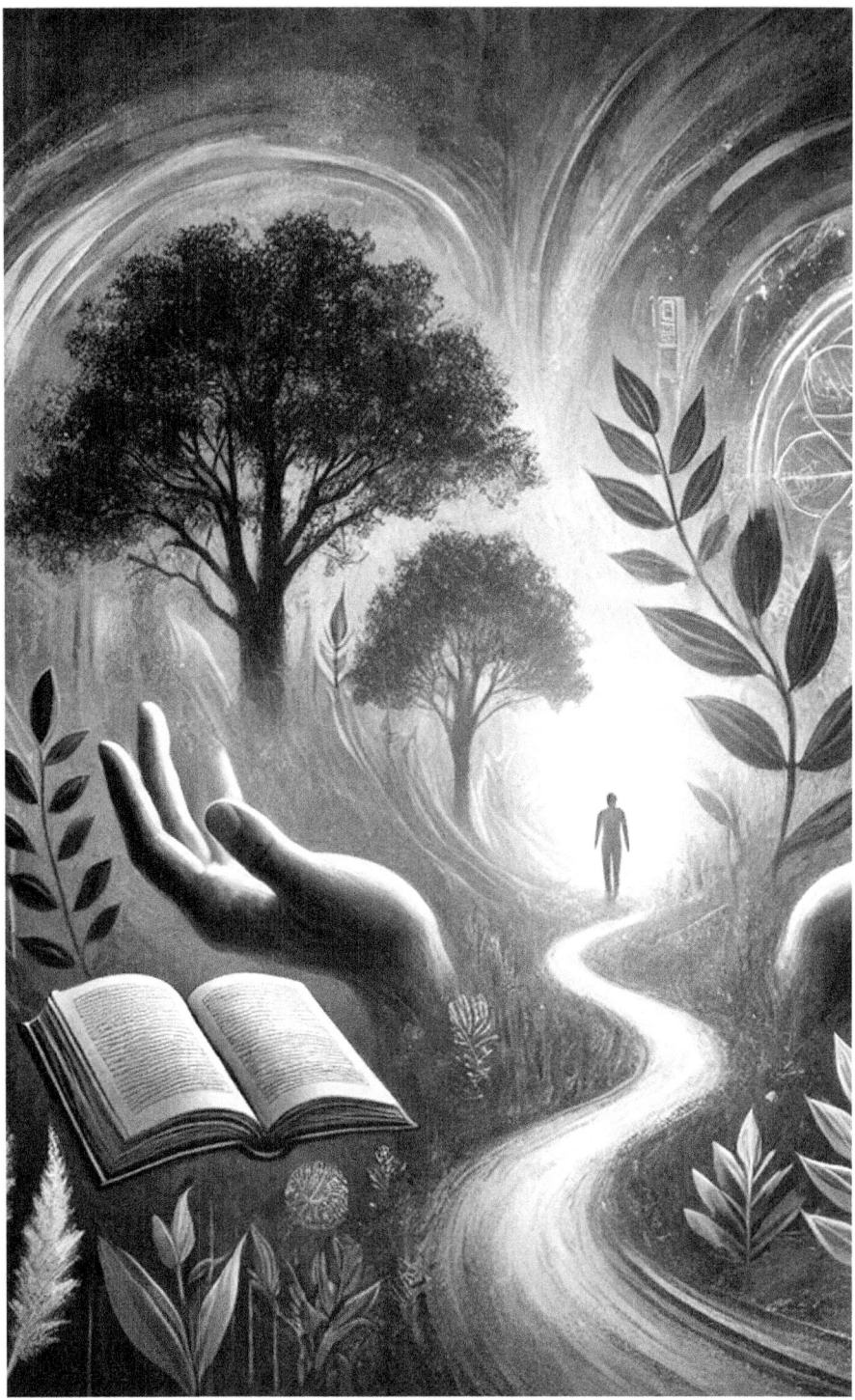

CHAPTER 3: SEEKING SCIENTIFIC APPROACHES TO CONFRONT CANCER – WISE DECISIONS AND CHOICES

After being discharged from the hospital, I made a heart-wrenching decision—to temporarily conceal the latest diagnosis from my family. They had been fully aware of my previous condition and had stood by me through waves of fear and disappointment. This time, however, I could not bear to drag them into the abyss of despair once more. My own state of mind was already in turmoil; adding their anxiety and pain would only make the burden even harder to bear. I realized that if they knew the harsh truth, their sense of helplessness and fear would mirror my own. Therefore, I chose to shoulder this pain alone, maintaining a façade of strength in their presence while fumbling through the darkness, desperately searching for a glimmer of hope.

Inside, my mind was a storm of chaos and anguish, as if swallowed by an all-encompassing void. I craved a moment of solitude—a quiet space where I could face the torrent of emotions surging within me and attempt to make sense of it all. Yet, the relentless urgency of time loomed like a sharpened blade, drawing closer with every passing moment. The shadow of death hung over me like an invisible shackle, pressing heavily on my chest, its weight suffocating and inescapable.

As the realization sank in that my life might soon come to an end, a wave of fear and sorrow crashed over me with overwhelming force. Once, I had thought these topics belonged to distant conversations about others, mere stories removed from my reality. But now, they were painfully close, tangible and inescapable. Every passing second brought a deep reflection on the meaning of life and an unprecedented sense of urgency: How much time do I have left? What will become of my unfulfilled dreams and unfinished plans? To my family and friends, I had always been a symbol of strength, but if they discovered the truth, how would they bear such a sudden and devastating blow? These questions swirled like a vortex in my mind, leaving me with a profound sense of loss and helplessness, as though my world had once again plunged into boundless turmoil and uncertainty.

Standing at the edge of fate's precipice, I was overwhelmed by an unparalleled sense of loneliness and grief, as though caught in a liminal space between life and death. The prospect of finding even a shred of hope became increasingly obscured. Though my body was back at home, my spirit felt directionless, lost, and unsure of the way forward. Confronted by this vast unknown, it was as if I had been cast into an infinite abyss, surrounded by impenetrable darkness. All I could do was inch forward with the utmost care, holding onto a faint flicker of hope. I longed for a single ray of light to pierce through the endless night, to guide me out of the oppressive gloom and illuminate a path toward renewal.

The Psychological Struggle: Finding Hope in the Midst of Despair

After enduring profound helplessness, my mind was torn by

countless internal conflicts and contradictions. I began to search for deeper meaning in the midst of this adversity, attempting to comprehend the essence of life and death and the possibilities that lie beyond them. This phase prompted unprecedented introspection into my life, relationships, and unfulfilled dreams. I reflected on my existence in this world, revisited every choice I had made, and contemplated the outcomes they had produced. Confronted with such a challenging situation, I understood that every action required careful deliberation. Identifying the best possible solution from the available options became crucial. Despite despair shadowing me at every turn, I remained lucid, knowing that recovery hinged on clear information and rational decisions.

Throughout surgery, chemotherapy, and radiotherapy, I endured nearly every imaginable side effect: changes in taste, nausea-induced appetite loss, and an inability to derive sufficient nutrition from the small amounts of food I could manage. Alternating episodes of diarrhea and constipation further compounded my physical distress. Doctors provided nutritional support and appetite stimulants, but these measures had little effect, and my condition showed almost no improvement. Meanwhile, depression, anxiety, and relentless stress weighed on me like an invisible burden, gradually eroding both my body and spirit.

During my hospital stay, I often felt like a product on an assembly line—processed swiftly and worn down in the process. My weight plummeted from nearly 90 kilograms to less than 50, leaving me emaciated to the point where "skin and bones" could barely describe my appearance. The astonished expressions of those who had once known me, upon seeing me again, remain seared in my memory. While I fully understood their reactions, they unwittingly added to my psychological burden, as the shadow of depression grew heavier over my heart. I frequently regretted not pursuing my dreams more fervently when I was healthy. At that moment, I realized that no amount of wealth could undo the mistakes of the past—life offers no medicine for regret. Yet, despite my internal struggles, I refused to give up on life. I chose to face my reality head-on and continued to explore every possible solution.

Even as my body grew weaker, I remained resolute, taking every step with determination. Although fear constantly hovered over me, my will to survive never faltered. Recognizing the importance of addressing reality, I resolved to use the time I had left to fulfill unfinished dreams, make peace with my past, and find inner tranquility. At the same time, I acknowledged the urgency of finding effective health management strategies in the face of advanced cancer. Time was of the essence, and I needed to make the wisest decisions without delay.

Cancer brings those of us who experience it not only physical torment but also profound uncertainty about the future and an acute awareness of life's fragility. Nevertheless, I refused to let these overwhelming emotions defeat me. I did not bow to the disease, nor did I relinquish my yearning for life. Gradually, I came to terms with my condition and began to delve into spiritual and philosophical questions, contemplating death, karma, the continuation of the soul, and the meaning of life. These thoughts surged through my mind like waves, returning again and again, leaving me restless yet reflective.

Eventually, I came to a profound realization: death is not the end of life but rather a transition, perhaps even a new beginning—an inevitable part of the journey. This new perspective brought me deep comfort and reignited a spark of hope within me. This spiritual awakening transformed my outlook on life, leading me to see that fighting cancer was not only about physical survival but also about redefining the value of life and the purpose of the struggle itself. This shift in mindset inspired me to explore alternative therapies and to believe that, with the right support, the body's natural ability to heal might be awakened and gradually strengthened.

Holding Onto Dreams: Resilience After Diagnosis

Before this diagnosis, I had many dreams and goals. Even in the face of such grim news, I refused to let go of them easily. While managing my business and overseeing a construction project, I made a conscious effort to spend quality time with my loved ones, engage in meaningful conversations, and express my wishes clearly to ensure they would be cared for, leaving behind cherished memories for us all. Although I often felt the pressing weight of time, I remained determined to pursue my unfulfilled aspirations, such as visiting places I had longed to see or completing my construction plans. To stay focused, I created a detailed to-do list, guiding me step by step toward these goals.

Throughout my battle, I kept myself extraordinarily busy, leaving little room to dwell on the possibility of my condition worsening. Looking back, I realize that staying occupied may have been a constructive coping mechanism. The demands of daily tasks temporarily distracted me from both physical and emotional pain. Working toward tangible goals gave me a renewed sense of control over my life, a feeling that had otherwise been slipping away.

I firmly believed that each day should be meaningful and fulfilling. This belief became the foundation for my courage to face the disease and embark on a new journey of exploration. I actively sought methods and resources to tap into my body's potential for self-healing, striving to find the most suitable path for my recovery. Even in moments of profound physical weakness, I continued to nourish my mind and soul, gradually building an inner strength. This intangible force propelled me forward, giving me the courage and motivation to rise against the odds.

One sleepless night, as I lay in bed overwhelmed by questions about my fate, I reflected on the moments of my life and silently prayed for more time to achieve my unrealized dreams. In that stillness, a voice echoed in my mind: "Do you want to keep living?" The question rang like a bell, reverberating deeply within me and bringing a sudden clarity. Time seemed to stand still as I pondered, and then, with unwavering resolve, I responded: "Yes, I want to live."

Looking back, this profound inner dialogue was far from coincidental. It reflected my positive mindset in the fight against illness and my strong will to survive. Perhaps it was nature's way of responding to my unwavering determination to live, or an internal dialogue sparked by a collision between my subconscious and conscious mind. I believe it was a manifestation of my agency actively influencing reality, or perhaps a psychological defense mechanism that helped me regain the motivation to keep fighting. Another possibility is that my deeply held belief system, core values, or innate survival instincts triggered a spiritual awakening or moment of enlightenment. Whatever the reason, from that moment onward, I felt a renewed yearning for life and made a firm decision to continue battling for survival.

Conventional medicine could no longer provide solutions for me, and the hospital had exhausted its options. In the days that followed, I gradually realized the urgency of taking immediate action—exploring every possible approach to extend my life and making the most rational decisions. Turning to alternative therapies became my only hope, a path I deeply felt was my last chance to continue living. Determined, I dedicated immense time and energy to thoroughly researching various strategies and methods, hoping to uncover an opportunity for survival.

Looking back, I understood that maintaining a positive mindset was absolutely essential. Even amidst intense suffering, I held onto my dreams and my desire to live. This conviction reinforced my belief in the power of the mind and the principles of attraction. To anyone fighting illness, my message is clear: even if doctors have given up, you must never abandon your faith in yourself. Without that belief, the answer is often final. After enduring eight months of pain, many may feel they no longer have the strength to keep going—but it is precisely in those moments that perseverance becomes most critical.

I had no examples of successful cancer survival around me, so I realized that knowledge was power. For those of us affected, gathering enough information is the only way to make the best possible decisions. Although despair and fear frequently loomed, I knew I was racing against time. In those critical moments, personal faith, mental strength, and love for my family and friends became the driving forces that kept me going.

With an open mind, I began exploring alternative therapies. Though my decision was difficult for others to understand, I firmly believed that I alone could be my best doctor and final hope. The path ahead was treacherous, but I moved forward without hesitation, convinced that my choices would ultimately lead me to recovery.

Knowledge is Power: Gathering Insights on Cancer

Beyond keeping myself extraordinarily busy, my strong will to survive and unwavering determination drove me to actively seek solutions rather than passively accept my fate. Resolute in my efforts to improve my chances of survival, I began to systematically gather research and information related to cancer, swiftly implementing various measures to explore potential strategies.

Through in-depth research, I delved into numerous health

management approaches, with a particular focus on alternative therapies. Utilizing online resources and other channels, I collected a vast amount of information from around the world on cancer management. I meticulously analyzed my condition and sought advice from multiple sources. During this period, reading articles, books, and scientific literature became a daily routine, while consultations with doctors and specialists deepened my understanding of potential approaches.

This process piqued my interest in alternative therapies and greatly motivated me to explore unconventional methods of support and treatment. After compiling extensive information on supportive and alternative therapies, I opted for an integrative health management approach. While it differed from conventional medical recommendations, this approach addressed not only physical recovery but also emotional, psychological, and spiritual well-being. It made me realize that my journey to recovery required taking greater personal responsibility.

By adopting this holistic strategy, I gradually reclaimed control over my recovery process and reignited a sense of hope. As I experimented with different recovery strategies, I continually adapted them to my unique needs, ensuring the best possible chances for healing. Although these efforts required time, they helped me better cope with physical changes, rebuild my confidence, and instilled in me a sense of forward momentum—a force propelling me through this challenging journey.

Emotional Anchor: Finding Warmth and Solace Within

Throughout my long battle with cancer, I chose not to reveal the harsh truth to my son. Perhaps it was parental instinct that drove me to shield him from the emotional pain and fear caused by my illness. I wanted to protect him from carrying such a heavy emotional burden at such a young age.

At just six years old, he lacked the capacity to fully comprehend the complexities of life, illness, and death. My concern was that such information might shatter his sense of security, disturb his inner peace, and hinder his psychological development and character formation. I feared that if he were unable to process and understand the gravity of the truth, it might leave lasting scars on his young heart. Thus, I worked hard to keep this harsh reality separate from his world, allowing him to enjoy as normal a childhood as possible. I refused to let the shadow of illness intrude upon his innocence and the beauty of his early years. My hope was for him to grow up carefree and joyful, unburdened by fear or unease caused by my condition.

While I actively sought treatments and explored alternative therapies, the uncertainty of the road ahead weighed heavily on my mind, weaving guilt and fear into the fabric of my thoughts. The decision to withhold the truth placed immense emotional and psychological pressure on me. I wrestled with the conflict between honesty and protection, trying to find the right moment and way to explain everything to him. Yet, I could never summon the courage, fearing the cascade of unpredictable emotional reactions that might follow. In many ways, this was a form of self-preservation—I avoided confronting a reality that would bring pain to both of us. Ultimately, I decided to keep the truth to myself for the time being.

I began cherishing every moment we spent together more than ever before. Each night, he would habitually hug me until I fell asleep before returning to his own room. This behavior was uncommon before my illness, but since then, he seemed to sense something instinctively. Though he never asked, his quiet suspicion and concern were evident, as if an unspoken intuition told him something significant was happening. I carefully maintained this precious bond, never hinting at the truth, unwilling to disrupt the fleeting peace and warmth of these moments.

Those nightly embraces became my greatest source of comfort and strength. I was acutely aware that I didn't know how long such happiness could last. Yet, his silent empathy and emotional sensitivity filled me with profound warmth and reminded me of his quiet growth. In the face of my overwhelming challenges, his dependence and care proved more therapeutic than any medicine, illuminating my days with hope. In the darkness of my struggles, his presence was like a warm light, dispelling the cold and giving me the courage to endure and move forward.

Conclusion

In this chapter, we delved into the profound psychological struggles and decision-making processes faced after a cancer diagnosis. For both individuals and their families, navigating the emotional spectrum between despair and hope is a delicate and often overwhelming challenge. Yet, even when the road ahead seems fraught with obstacles, the desire for recovery must not be abandoned. By deepening our understanding of cancer and exploring various strategies for coping, we can empower ourselves to make more informed and rational choices. It is unwavering faith that becomes a formidable force, enabling us to keep moving forward in the face of adversity.

Upon receiving a prognosis that quantified the time I might have left, I chose to act immediately, seeking a broader and more comprehensive path to recovery. This journey led me to explore alternative therapies as a means to complement and expand the reach of conventional treatments. Along the way, I found my confidence gradually rekindled. A positive mindset, coupled with the relentless pursuit of unfulfilled dreams, became the foundation for overcoming inner despair. These elements infused my life with a renewed sense of purpose and vitality, proving that even in the darkest moments, hope and determination can pave the way to resilience and growth.

CHUNMEI YAO

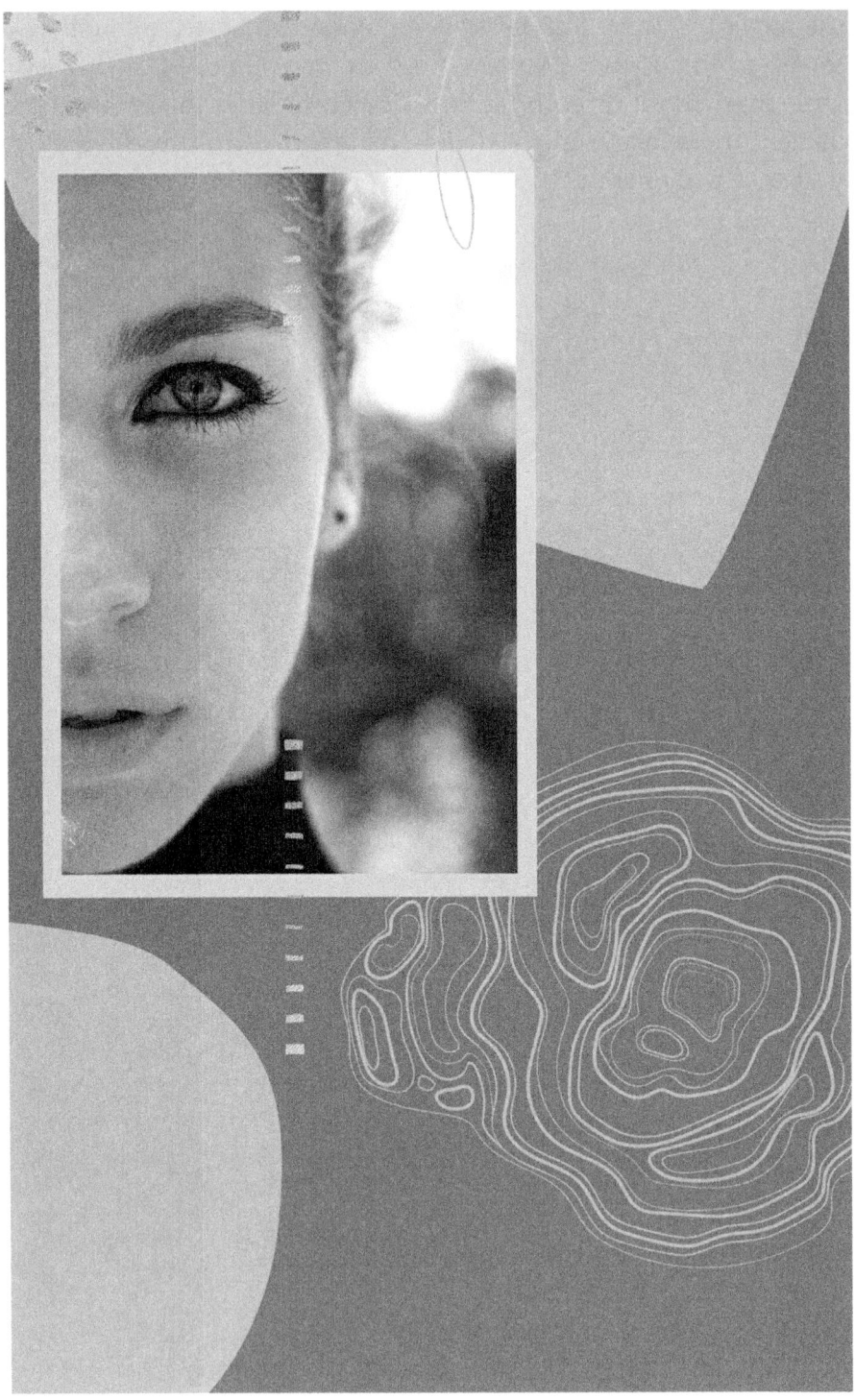

CHAPTER 4: THE JOURNEY OF CONQUERING CANCER – A GUIDE TO SELF-RECONSTRUCTION

In the previous chapter, we delved into the profound psychological struggles and critical decision-making faced when confronting cancer, emphasizing how understanding essential information and cultivating unwavering belief can ignite the strength to move forward even in moments of despair. However, the true journey of overcoming cancer begins here. Grasping these concepts is merely the starting point; the true challenge lies in integrating them into daily life—a demanding yet pivotal endeavor.

This chapter takes us to the starting line of this battle, exploring how to bravely embark on the path of holistic self-reconstruction. When physical and emotional exhaustion pushed me to the brink of collapse, and the side effects of treatments relentlessly eroded my body, leading to progressive liver and kidney dysfunction, I found myself trapped in a vicious cycle exacerbated by sleep disturbances and impaired detoxification. This invisible drain dragged me into the depths of despair, allowing me to profoundly grasp the meaning of being at rock bottom.

Amid this turmoil, I made a life-altering decision: to embrace alternative therapies and embark on a new journey toward comprehensive recovery. Despite the uncertainties ahead, especially in the face of limited improvements from conventional medicine, I chose to proceed with courage. As I gradually uncovered the potential of alternative treatments, I realized that genuine recovery goes beyond medical interventions. It requires a holistic approach to healing—one that harmonizes the body, mind, and spirit to restore inner balance and well-being.

This chapter recounts the critical first steps I took to discover new hope and breakthroughs, exploring and uncovering my own path to holistic health. Throughout this challenging journey, I experienced the transformative power of self-reconstruction, ultimately finding the courage to seek the miracle of recovery.

Alternative Therapies: Expectations and Challenges

In the early stages of my journey, I vividly felt the immense toll cancer cells took on my physical strength. My body was frequently overwhelmed by extreme fatigue, as the battle against cancer drained my energy reserves and intensified a persistent sense of exhaustion. With diminished appetite and poor nutrient absorption, my strength failed to recover, leaving me feeling increasingly frail. To make matters worse, prolonged insomnia exacerbated my suffering, intensifying pain and stress to the point where I felt both my body and spirit were crushed under an unbearable weight.

The emotional burden was equally significant. Despite my best efforts to maintain a positive outlook, anxiety and depression lingered like relentless shadows, eroding my mental resilience and hindering my recovery. As my physical condition deteriorated, the imbalance in my sympathetic nervous system deepened my fatigue. Facing an uncertain future, I often felt isolated and overwhelmed by a profound sense of helplessness and unease.

As I explored alternative therapies, I gradually realized that recovery required more than physical effort; it also depended on mental fortitude and emotional equilibrium. These therapies not only facilitated progress in restoring my physical and emotional well-being but also taught me valuable strategies for coping with life's challenges and pressures. Alternative therapies encompass various approaches, including herbal remedies, physical exercises, and stress management techniques, showing remarkable effectiveness in alleviating treatment side effects. Through these methods, I managed to reduce nausea, vomiting, anemia, and pain. As my emotions stabilized, I regained a sense of control over my health.

However, maintaining realistic expectations during the initial stages of alternative therapy proved crucial. I naively hoped for immediate results, only to quickly realize that the benefits of these treatments required time and patience to manifest. Each individual's body responds differently, and finding the right approach to health management often involves ongoing experimentation and adjustment. This journey, while filled with uncertainties, taught me the importance of perseverance and patience as I navigated the path forward.

As my body gradually adapted to these therapeutic interventions, my immune system began to regain balance, enhancing my ability to resist cancer cells. Although the journey was fraught with challenges, I held onto the belief that perseverance and effort would eventually bring a glimmer of hope, allowing me to reclaim control over the course of my life.

Managing Side Effects: Practical Strategies

During the initial phase of alternative therapy, the body often requires time to adapt to newly introduced elements and holistic treatment approaches. I gradually came to understand the importance of implementing comprehensive and targeted support measures. These not only helped alleviate discomfort during the adaptation process but also ensured the smooth progression of the entire treatment. As previously mentioned, individual responses to alternative therapies can vary significantly. In the first few weeks or even months, fluctuations in symptoms, emotional swings, or unstable physical reactions are natural adjustment responses and an inevitable part of the recovery journey.

I opted for a gradual introduction of new health management practices rather than making abrupt and extensive changes all at once. This gentle transition gave my body sufficient time to adjust, reducing the likelihood of severe reactions or discomfort. Listening to my body's feedback became crucial—by closely monitoring the effects of different therapies, I could promptly adjust my recovery plan to minimize adverse effects. At the same time, I prioritized rest and relaxation, avoiding overexertion to better equip my body to handle the stress of treatment.

In addressing side effects, I discovered several effective practical strategies. First and foremost, maintaining adequate daily hydration proved essential, as it not only facilitated detoxification but also improved overall health. Second, ensuring a balanced diet helped strengthen my immune system, making my body more resilient to the challenges posed by treatment. Additionally, sufficient and high-quality sleep emerged as a cornerstone of recovery, playing a vital role in the body's natural healing processes. The critical roles of hydration, nutrition, detoxification, and sleep in this journey will be explored in greater detail in the following chapter.

With these lifestyle adjustments, I began to notice a gradual reduction in adverse reactions and a corresponding improvement in overall health. As my body's resilience increased, I found myself better equipped to face the challenges of illness with greater strength and determination. Each small step toward restoring balance not only reinforced my confidence but also underscored the profound impact even minor changes can have on the path to recovery.

These practical management strategies helped me navigate the adjustment period of alternative therapy while fostering a deeper awareness and respect for my body's needs. Through this journey, I developed a flexible and intuitive mindset, allowing me to adapt my approach as circumstances evolved. This heightened awareness not only enabled me to better endure the treatment but also helped me rediscover the vitality of life, providing an unwavering source of strength as I continued forward.

Overcoming Setbacks: A Journey of Ups and Downs

These therapies typically avoid the use of chemical drugs, resulting in milder side effects and gentler physical responses. However, occasional mild discomfort is to be expected. Such reactions, often referred to as "self-regulation responses," are common manifestations of the body's adaptation and self-adjustment processes. As the treatment progresses and the body gradually acclimates, these discomforts tend to subside, helping to foster greater confidence in managing my health.

Regardless of the therapy chosen, setbacks are an inherent part of the process. At times, symptoms may temporarily worsen, new discomforts may arise, or certain therapies may fail to deliver the anticipated improvements. Yet, these fluctuations do not signify a dead end in the recovery journey; they are often natural responses during the body's adjustment phase. What matters most is maintaining a positive outlook and preparing mentally to embrace these ups and downs as integral components of the healing process. The interplay between physical responses and psychological challenges weaves together the fabric of this tumultuous yet transformative journey.

When setbacks occur, the ability to adapt and adjust strategies becomes crucial. The unwavering support and encouragement of family and friends, combined with my own hope for the future, served as a source of strength during difficult times. It is essential to remember that progress from illness to health is rarely a straight line; it often resembles a winding mountain road, with moments of advancement, pauses, and even occasional regressions. Much like the trajectory of life itself, there are peaks and valleys. Each setback carries the potential for growth, and overcoming these fluctuations brings me one step closer to the ultimate goal of recovery.

Perseverance and flexibility have been the keys to sustaining my journey forward. As my body gradually adapted, my condition began to stabilize, marking not only a profound test of my mental resilience but also a vital stage of the recovery process. On this path, only by balancing determination with adaptability can one witness the gradual emergence of therapeutic benefits and ultimately reach the shores of restored health.

Resilience and Perseverance: Driving Forces During Recovery

Resilience, the capacity to remain steadfast and recover in the face of adversity, is particularly crucial during the early stages of recovery. It not only helps us withstand successive setbacks but also fuels the drive to keep moving forward. No matter how daunting the challenges may seem, resilience keeps us focused on our recovery goals, preventing us from giving up and often strengthening our resolve with each setback. By continually cultivating this quality, we equip ourselves to overcome illness and lay a solid foundation for pursuing a healthier, more fulfilling life.

For individuals affected by late-stage cancer, these therapies often require an extended timeline, and choosing this path demands immense courage and determination. Amid physical pain and inner struggles, resilience emerges as the core strength that enables us to confront uncertainties and challenges. With unwavering faith and an indomitable spirit, we navigate this thorn-filled recovery journey with dignity, face each obstacle with determination, and embrace the future with a hopeful heart.

During recovery, maintaining a balanced mindset—one that confronts reality while holding onto hope—is vital. Though the path to recovery is often filled with ups and downs, optimism can unlock our inner potential, helping us find the strength to move forward. As the body gradually adapts and adjusts, resilience grows stronger, steadily paving the way toward ultimate healing and bringing with it the first glimmers of hope.

Resilience is not just a psychological anchor but an indispensable source of spiritual strength throughout the recovery process. Through unwavering perseverance and adaptive responses, we can find our rhythm amid the fluctuations of recovery and progress steadily with confidence. Each act of perseverance brings us closer to the goal of recovery. Ultimately, through countless trials and moments of growth, we will achieve the goal of healing and rediscover the power of a renewed life.

Conclusion

This chapter has delved into the multifaceted challenges encountered during the early stages of battling cancer, emphasizing the need for a comprehensive approach to address both physical adaptation and mental resilience. Through the exploration of alternative therapies, we have come to understand that each recovery journey is unique. Alternative therapies represent more than a choice—they symbolize the courageous first step toward discovery. Along this path, the uncertainties and potential challenges posed by these therapies are inevitable, making the process of overcoming them a vital part of the recovery experience.

When managing the side effects of treatment, practical and proven strategies have been shown to provide significant support. Thoughtful, detailed measures create a strong foundation for physical recovery, helping us to actively navigate discomfort and offering valuable, tangible assistance in alleviating the hardships of treatment.

Facing setbacks in recovery requires an unwavering belief in the possibility of healing. Resilience serves as the cornerstone for overcoming obstacles on this journey. By progressively strengthening this quality, we can persevere through the processes of recovery and self-reconstruction, gradually adapting to physical and psychological changes while confronting new challenges with determination.

In summary, this chapter highlights the importance of moving forward with both courage and adaptability in this often unpredictable health management journey. Through an integrated strategy and a steadfast will, we are able to progress steadily, continuously adjusting to face each twist and turn of the future. Along this path, a resolute spirit and the ability to adapt become inexhaustible sources of strength, driving us forward toward recovery and renewal.

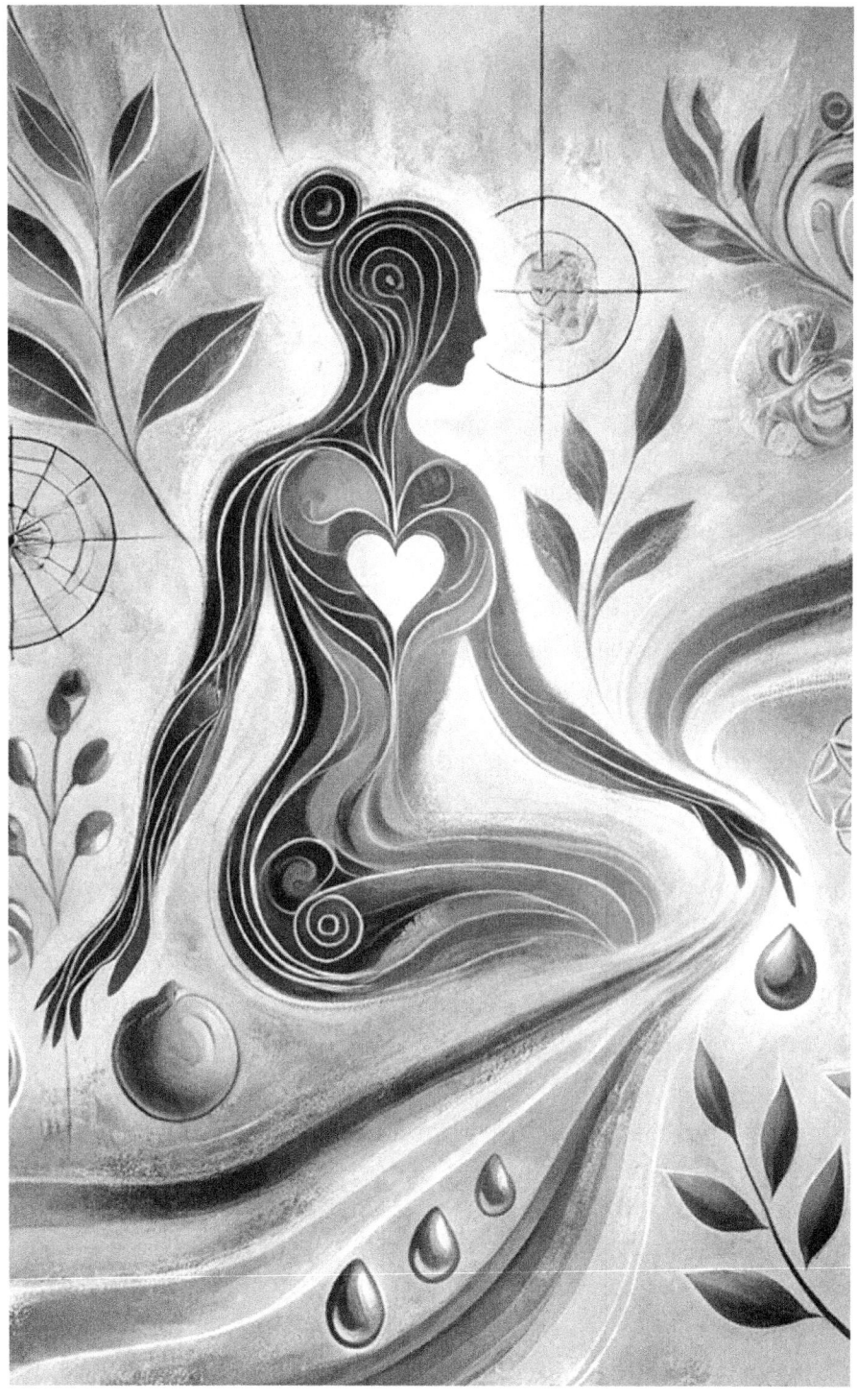

CHAPTER 5: UNLOCKING THE BODY'S HEALING POTENTIAL – WISDOM AND PRACTICE

In the previous chapter, we explored the psychological preparedness required when adopting alternative therapies, strategies for managing potential side effects, and the critical role of resilience throughout the process. Maintaining mental fortitude amid the challenges and setbacks posed by illness is undoubtedly a key driver of physical recovery. During this journey, a positive, constructive mindset provided robust support for my body's healing process, not only strengthening my emotional resilience but also instilling greater confidence to face each day's trials.

This chapter delves deeper into how alternative therapies can unlock the body's innate healing potential, paving the way for comprehensive recovery and ultimately overcoming illness. As my understanding of alternative therapies grew, I began to feel a greater sense of control over my health, reinforcing my determination to combat the disease.

Through continued practice, I gradually realized that conquering cancer requires more than external interventions—it also demands active self-care to accelerate the recovery process. By making lifestyle adjustments and setting achievable, incremental goals, I observed steady progress in my daily life. These small victories boosted my sense of accomplishment, bolstered my confidence in the overall process, and injected positive momentum into my recovery, laying a solid foundation for achieving long-term health.

As part of this journey, I also incorporated homeopathy into my regimen. This individualized and holistic approach allowed me to tailor treatments to my specific needs. A form of alternative medicine, homeopathy emphasizes the use of highly diluted natural substances and relies on the body's inherent healing capabilities. While scientific studies suggest that its effects may primarily stem from a placebo response, I, like many other practitioners, experienced tangible and positive changes. At that stage, the effectiveness of the treatment mattered most to me, and homeopathy provided valuable support in this regard.

Ultimately, my choice of these methods was not solely aimed at extending my life but also at enhancing its quality and meaning. The courage to explore diverse health strategies and the steadfast belief in their potential benefits became vital pillars supporting me through this transformative journey.

My Comprehensive Cancer Recovery Strategy: From Theory to Practice

Adopting alternative therapies was not merely a hopeful choice for me but also a journey of exploration and overcoming challenges. A personalized recovery plan addressed not only my physical healing needs but also supported emotional and mental balance, seamlessly integrating into my daily routine. This approach ensured continuity throughout the process while progressively improving my quality of life. The flexibility of alternative therapies allowed me to continuously adjust and optimize my treatments based on my body's responses, enabling me to find the most suitable approach and lay a solid foundation for restoring overall health.

During this journey, certain therapies proved effective not only in alleviating physical discomfort but also in gradually restoring harmony between my body and mind. While these therapies generally had mild effects, they occasionally caused side effects, such as allergic reactions or potential drug interactions. To ensure safety, I always started with small doses, carefully monitored my body's reactions, and promptly adjusted my recovery plan if any abnormalities arose. Through long-term practice and adjustments, these methods evolved into a comprehensive health system. My decisions consistently drew from extensive research, supported by a wealth of scientific literature and medical resources.

The remarkable advantage of alternative therapies lies in their holistic approach. They focus not only on symptom management but also on enhancing overall well-being, activating the body's innate healing potential. By employing this comprehensive recovery strategy, I gradually regained confidence in life, significantly strengthening my immune system and improving my physical condition.

The most valuable lesson I learned along the way is that caution, flexibility, continuous learning, and consistent adjustment are essential to finding therapies that truly work for you. The recovery journey is a testament to perseverance and unwavering belief, driven by the relentless pursuit of balance and health for both the mind and body.

Here are the strategies I adopted, which together provided comprehensive support on my journey to overcoming cancer and helped me successfully navigate various challenges. I hope these approaches can offer you valuable assistance and inspiration during difficult times.

Improving the Sleep

Environment: A Crucial Factor in Fighting Cancer

As discussed in Chapter 4, high-quality sleep is essential for the body's self-repair and can mitigate the side effects of chemotherapy or radiation therapy. Moreover, sleep plays a crucial role in supporting immune system function, regulating hormone levels, and enhancing psychological resilience—all of which are vital factors in the fight against cancer. This section focuses on optimizing the sleep environment to amplify these positive effects, balancing personal energy and electromagnetic fields, and significantly improving sleep quality to promote recovery effectively.

Enhancing the sleep environment not only improves energy flow, magnetic balance, and sleep quality but also elevates overall sensory experiences, creates a more soothing atmosphere, and contributes to a sense of well-being. This explains why certain spaces feel calming, while others may evoke unease or tension. Some environments may accumulate negative energy due to magnetic field anomalies or other factors, affecting the occupant's mood, sleep quality, and ultimately, health. Uncomfortable spaces often harbor such negative energies. A crucial step in improving the sleep environment is to isolate and eliminate these potentially harmful energy fields, enabling a more positive mindset to confront illness.

Optimizing the sleep environment can significantly impact physical regeneration and immune system function. By adjusting the surroundings, energy flow can be facilitated, better supporting the body's recovery process. While some may remain skeptical about these practices, I firmly believe that these adjustments have had a positive effect on my recovery.

For me, improving the sleep environment—and by extension, my living environment—was a critical aspect of my cancer recovery journey. Our living spaces are not merely three-dimensional constructs; from a metaphysical perspective, the universe comprises multiple dimensions, including dark matter and dark energy. What we perceive is just a fraction of the whole, and the unseen elements often have a decisive impact on our health. Their invisibility does not negate their existence.

Understanding these dimensions complements other therapies and serves as an indispensable element of recovery, as quality sleep provides a solid foundation for overall health. In the early stages of my journey, I made comprehensive changes to my sleep environment: I moved into a sunlit room, replaced my bed and bedding, and minimized potential harmful factors, creating a supportive space for my recovery.

If your sleeping space is limited, even small adjustments—such as repositioning your bed, reorienting its placement, or replacing bedding—can provide significant benefits. These seemingly simple changes could yield unexpected positive effects on your recovery and overall well-being.

Key Guidelines for Adjusting Bed Placement to Enhance Health, Energy Flow, and Recovery

1. Position the Headboard Against a Solid Wall

The headboard should rest against a sturdy wall to symbolize stability and a sense of security. Avoid placing the headboard near windows or open spaces, as this can create a lack of support and a feeling of vulnerability, leaving you more susceptible to external disturbances or cold drafts, which may negatively impact health. If the room layout limits your options, consider using heavy curtains, adding a headboard, or placing a screen to counteract the negative effects of a window behind the bed, thereby improving sleep quality and promoting positive energy.

2. Avoid Aligning the Foot of the Bed with the Door

In traditional feng shui, positioning the foot of the bed directly in line with the door is referred to as the "coffin position," which is believed to invite negative energy or unfavorable outcomes. If rearranging the bed is not feasible, you can mitigate this by using a screen or hanging a curtain to block the view of the door, reducing potential adverse effects on health.

3. Keep the Bed Away from Beams Overhead

Avoid placing the bed directly beneath exposed beams, as this creates a feeling of pressure and may disrupt sleep, adversely affecting health. If unavoidable, consider mitigating this effect with ceiling modifications or by using a canopy bed. Canopies can range from light, airy drapes to heavier fabrics, combining aesthetic appeal with functionality to minimize the impact of overhead beams.

4. Avoid Mirrors Facing the Bed

Mirrors that face the bed can reflect energy, disrupting sleep and impacting health. This is particularly problematic at night, as waking up to see a distorted reflection may cause fear or psychological stress. If removing the mirror is not possible, use curtains, covers, or a screen to block the mirror, preventing energy reflection and creating a more peaceful sleep environment.

5. Avoid Aligning the Bed with Bathrooms or Kitchens

The dampness of bathrooms and the heat from kitchens can introduce negative elements into the bedroom, affecting air quality and disrupting energy flow. Over time, these factors may harm health and reduce sleep quality, impacting overall physical and mental balance.

6. Ensure Good Ventilation Around the Bed

Proper air circulation in the bedroom is essential for energy flow. Keeping the room well-ventilated not only introduces fresh air but also fosters positive energy, creating a healthier environment conducive to restful sleep.

7. Keep the Area Under the Bed Clutter-Free

Avoid storing items under the bed to maintain cleanliness and prevent blocked energy flow. Accumulated clutter can attract dust and negative energy, which may harm physical and mental health. Keeping the space beneath the bed clear promotes better air circulation and establishes a harmonious sleep environment.

8. Minimize Exposure to Electromagnetic Interference

To improve sleep quality, place the bed away from electronic devices such as TVs, computers, and phone chargers, as the electromagnetic fields they emit may disrupt the body's natural balance. Wireless devices like routers should be positioned away from the bedroom or turned off at night. Avoid keeping phones, tablets, or other electronics near the bed. If necessary, place them at a distance or switch them to airplane mode to reduce electromagnetic exposure and foster a quieter, distraction-free environment.

9. Consider Bed Orientation

Traditional beliefs suggest that aligning the body's magnetic field with the Earth's magnetic field promotes balance and well-being. Generally, positioning the headboard to face north or east is considered optimal for aligning with the Earth's geomagnetic direction, promoting restful sleep and emotional stability. Alternatively, selecting an orientation that feels personally comfortable may also yield positive psychological effects.

By following these principles and adjustments, you can effectively reduce disruptions to your sleep environment, optimize energy flow, and support physical and mental recovery. While these changes may seem simple, integrating feng shui concepts and minimizing electromagnetic interference can significantly improve energy dynamics, contributing to better overall health.

Ultimately, these modifications not only optimize the physical aspects of the sleeping environment but also enhance the symbolic and psychological factors that influence well-being. Through these efforts, you can foster an environment conducive to faster and more effective recovery.

The specific reasons and effects of changing my sleep environment are as follows:

1. Feng Shui and Health

Feng Shui emphasizes the profound impact of environmental harmony on health. By rearranging the placement of rooms and beds, it is possible to optimize energy flow, thereby enhancing physical and mental well-being. Feng Shui theory suggests that a clean and well-organized small bedroom is more likely to "gather energy," preventing it from dispersing and helping to create a stable and peaceful energy field. The compact nature of a small bedroom also provides a sense of enclosure, offering residents a feeling of safety and comfort, which in turn promotes physical and mental balance. Therefore, Feng Shui emphasizes the principle of "capturing and retaining energy." By maintaining a tidy environment and optimizing the layout—such as the positioning of the bed and the introduction of natural light—the gathering of energy can be further enhanced.

A clean and organized space not only supports the accumulation of positive energy while avoiding the stagnation of negative energy but also facilitates the free flow of energy, reducing obstructions and fostering a harmonious and balanced living environment. Moreover, such an environment positively impacts psychological well-being, aiding in the restoration of inner energy balance. It is evident that a clean and orderly living space not only enhances physical comfort but also improves mental state, ultimately contributing to health, happiness, and success.

In conclusion, the idea that "a small bedroom can gather energy" represents a combination of Feng Shui principles on energy concentration and environmental psychology. It serves not only to meet the practical demands of comfortable living but also reflects the profound cultural pursuit of balance between space and energy flow in traditional Feng Shui.

2. Integration of Magnetic Field Theory and Feng Shui

From the perspective of magnetic field theory, the Earth's magnetic field and electromagnetic fields may influence human health. Alternative medicine suggests that negative energy or electromagnetic interference can undermine health. By adjusting the sleep environment and positioning, such interference can be minimized, purifying the surroundings and enhancing energy fields, ultimately creating favorable conditions for restorative sleep.

Magnetic field theory and Feng Shui stem from different traditions but share a common emphasis on the environment's impact on health and well-being. Feng Shui, a Chinese practice with over 3,000 years of history, draws upon ancient Chinese philosophies, geography, architecture, and cosmology to optimize the flow of energy (Qi) within a space to achieve harmony, prosperity, and health. In practical applications, Feng Shui occasionally incorporates knowledge of magnetic fields to identify the optimal energy flow direction within a room, further enhancing the environment's positive effects on physical and psychological health.

3. The Metaphysical Perspective

As part of traditional Chinese mysticism, metaphysics explores the relationship between humans, nature, and the universe. Within this context, changes to sleep positioning and bedding symbolize the initiation of an energy purification and healing process. These adjustments not only help rebalance the energy field but also provide psychological support and motivation, fostering emotional and psychological recovery.

4. Psychology and Symbolism

Altering the room and bedding also holds symbolic significance, representing a fresh start and helping discard old negative and harmful associations. This transformation creates a new environment conducive to recovery. Such changes not only bring a sense of psychological renewal but also enhance mental strength, helping to cultivate a more positive mindset to confront illness, thereby effectively supporting physical recovery.

5. The Power of Belief

Improving the sleep environment can bring about positive psychological and emotional changes while strengthening the power of belief and reinforcing positive psychological suggestions. This effect is closely tied to energy fields. Thus, optimizing the living environment can help individuals experience peace and tranquility. When surrounded by positive energy, the body's healing process is positively influenced, accelerating the journey to recovery.

In alternative therapies, belief is considered a key factor in the healing process. By enhancing the environment, positive beliefs are cultivated, explaining why belief is often regarded as a significant auxiliary force in many health management strategies. While belief itself cannot directly cure diseases, it can activate the body's self-healing mechanisms, such as promoting the release of endorphins, resulting in tangible physiological and psychological effects. These effects include alleviating pain, improving mood, enhancing mental state, reducing stress, and boosting immune function, thereby supporting gradual overall health recovery.

This outcome is similar to the placebo effect mentioned earlier in this chapter regarding homeopathy. Studies have shown that the placebo effect not only applies to interventions with no specific therapeutic effect but also facilitates positive health improvements through psychological suggestion and mind-body interaction, thereby amplifying the effectiveness of various coping strategies.

In summary, these changes represent an effective alternative therapy, integrating environmental, physical, psychological, and energetic factors to enhance overall health comprehensively. These adjustments not only improve the sensory impact of the external environment but also provide strong psychological support for physical recovery, enabling me to maintain a positive mindset and good spirits throughout the healing process.

Detoxification: The Core of Health and Recovery

Upon embarking on my journey of self-regulation, I gradually realized that detoxification is regarded as having a certain role in some holistic therapies. It is considered a step that helps the body eliminate unnecessary metabolic byproducts, supporting its normal functions. By detoxifying, the functions of vital organs such as the liver and kidneys can be enhanced, allowing them to operate more efficiently. The accumulation of metabolic byproducts may impact the performance of the digestive, absorption, and excretory systems.

In such cases, nutrients may not be fully absorbed and could even place an additional burden on the body.

Adopting healthy lifestyle habits enables the body to better maintain its self-repair mechanisms and improve the efficiency of nutrient absorption. As vitality is gradually restored, immune function is supported, laying the groundwork for subsequent natural therapies and becoming a vital component of the recovery process.

I deeply understand that eliminating metabolic byproducts is not only a starting point for physical recovery but also a critical factor in supporting overall health. In the early stages of my self-regulation, focusing on enhancing detoxification played a positive role, while various nutrients in my diet proved indispensable during this process. A healthy diet acts as a natural cleanser, helping the body maintain metabolic balance and providing the necessary nutrients to ensure proper functioning. Nutrient-rich meals help the liver, kidneys, digestive system, and immune system work more efficiently, supporting metabolic balance, enhancing the body's self-repair capabilities, and boosting overall vitality.

Moreover, healthy dietary habits can improve sleep quality, and deep sleep aids in daily repair and metabolic balance. Research indicates that only during deep sleep do brain neurons fully rest and complete daily metabolism, which explains why high-quality sleep leaves one refreshed and energetic the next day.

The close connection between sleep and gut health cannot be overlooked either. Sleep deprivation may lead to an imbalance in gut microbiota, which, in turn, can further affect sleep quality. This interplay highlights the importance of maintaining a healthy lifestyle for everyone, especially for individuals affected by cancer. Deep sleep is not only a critical stage for physical repair but also provides an optimal opportunity for recovery. The gut, as one of the body's key detoxification pathways, works in conjunction with the liver and kidneys to help eliminate waste, thereby supporting overall health.

Additionally, to achieve better sleep, one may consider consuming a small amount of food before bedtime while maintaining a slight sense of hunger. This can enhance the quality of deep sleep and stimulate the body's self-healing abilities and immunity. This wisdom about sleep originates from the Huangdi Neijing (The Yellow Emperor's Inner Canon), showcasing the profound understanding of health in ancient times.

During the process of addressing cancer, the immune system may be affected to some extent. Maintaining good nutritional intake helps balance and support immune function. Through detoxification and adequate nutrient intake, inflammation in the body can be alleviated, supporting the immune system's balance and normal function. This, in turn, accelerates the recovery process and enhances overall health.

In summary, adequate nutrition is key to supporting the body's natural detoxification functions. In alternative medicine and the field of health, this concept of promoting detoxification through a healthy diet is widely recognized. In the following chapters, we will explore this topic in greater detail.

Here are several effective detoxification methods, particularly in terms of dietary strategies, which form a central component of physical recovery.

Chlorella, Spirulina, And Kelp: Detoxification And Health Support

Organic chlorella, spirulina, and kelp are nutrient-rich algae belonging to the categories of green algae, blue-green algae, and brown algae, respectively. They are highly regarded for their unique nutritional profiles and extensive health benefits. Additionally, this chapter will introduce another type of algae—red algae. Together with green, blue-green, and brown algae, red algae constitute the broader classification of "algae." These algae share the ability to perform photosynthesis, thrive in aquatic environments, and serve similar roles within ecosystems.

Chlorella is particularly effective in detoxification, spirulina is renowned for its high protein content and antioxidant properties, and kelp is rich in minerals, especially iodine, which supports thyroid function. Together, they provide a wealth of vitamins, minerals, and antioxidants that can effectively enhance overall health and support the immune system.

The detailed explanations are as follows:

1. Chlorella: A Natural Detoxifier

Chlorella, a nutrient-dense freshwater green algae, has garnered attention for its potential detoxifying and anticancer properties. It is rich in high-quality proteins, vitamins, minerals, and antioxidants, providing comprehensive nutritional support to the body. The cell walls of chlorella contain polysaccharides and cellulose, which bind to and eliminate harmful substances like heavy metals, earning it the title of a "natural detoxifier."

2. Spirulina: High-Protein and Antioxidant Support

Spirulina, a blue-green algae, boasts a protein content of 60-70% and contains all essential amino acids required by the human body. It is packed with beta-carotene, B vitamins, iron, calcium, magnesium, and antioxidant compounds such as phycocyanin, which help neutralize free radicals, slow cellular aging, and bolster the immune system. Additionally, spirulina promotes bile secretion, aiding liver detoxification and optimizing digestive system function.

3. Kelp: Natural Support for Minerals and Thyroid Health

Kelp, a large seaweed, is renowned for its detoxifying properties and is rich in iodine, fiber, vitamin K, folate, and various minerals, including calcium, magnesium, and iron. Its fucoidans and antioxidants provide significant benefits for cardiovascular health and immune function. Kelp's absorptive properties make it an excellent natural detoxifier, especially for removing heavy metals and radioactive substances. It also positively impacts bone, dental, and cardiovascular health.

4. Comprehensive Benefits: Complementary Detoxification and Nutritional Support

Chlorella binds to toxins within the body through its cell wall components and aids in their elimination, while kelp, with its adsorption properties, assists in the removal of harmful substances. When consumed together, these two superfoods provide complementary nutritional benefits—combining the proteins and chlorophyll in chlorella with the iodine and minerals found in kelp. This synergy helps maintain energy levels, strengthen immunity, and support the body's natural detoxification processes.

Incorporating these algae into a recovery-focused daily diet can provide thorough detoxification for the body. Their unique synergistic properties effectively boost the immune system, supply essential nutrients, and support recovery while enhancing vitality and overall well-being.

In summary, chlorella, spirulina, and kelp work together to provide comprehensive nutrition, detoxification, and enhanced health support. Chlorella removes toxins and supplies trace elements, spirulina contributes high-quality protein and antioxidant properties that bolster immunity and combat aging, and kelp replenishes minerals, supports thyroid health, and maintains metabolic balance. Combined, these three algae form an integrated health support system, offering deep nutrition and detoxification assistance. They are an ideal choice for promoting overall health and serving as a complementary therapy in cancer care.

Vegetable And Fruit Juices: Natural Detoxification

Detoxifying vegetable and fruit juices are made by blending a variety of nutrient-rich vegetables and fruits using a juicer or blender. These juices are packed with vitamins, minerals, and antioxidants that not only support the function of vital organs such as the liver and kidneys to enhance the body's detoxification capacity but also play a significant role in promoting cancer recovery.

The antioxidants in vegetable and fruit juices can help neutralize free radicals in the body, reducing cellular damage caused by oxidative stress, which plays an important role in preventing the transformation of normal cells into cancerous ones. Incorporating whole fruits and vegetables, including their pulp and dietary fiber, helps retain their full nutritional value. Dietary fiber gently supports intestinal peristalsis, aids digestion and waste elimination, and binds to harmful substances in the gut, assisting their removal and reducing the reabsorption of toxins. This process contributes to better intestinal health. Additionally, dietary fiber naturally extends the feeling of fullness and helps maintain stable blood sugar levels, offering a more balanced and nourishing approach to health.

Moreover, the diverse nutrients in these juices significantly boost the immune system, helping the body better resist external harmful factors and internal physiological changes. By providing the body with a concentrated dose of nutrients, vegetable and fruit juices improve nutritional intake efficiency while reducing the burden on digestion and absorption, thereby supporting faster recovery. This comprehensive nutritional support makes detoxifying vegetable and fruit juices an essential component in enhancing overall health and improving recovery outcomes.

Below are some of the combinations I frequently use during this period, which have proven to be highly effective. You can also adapt them flexibly based on your individual needs, tastes, and preferences.

1. Spinach + Cucumber + Apple + Lemon

This combination is refreshing and energizing, particularly beneficial for supporting kidney health and the digestive system. Spinach is rich in vitamins A, C, and K, as well as iron, helping to eliminate free radicals and enhance liver detoxification. However, spinach contains oxalic acid, which is readily absorbed by the body and can interfere with calcium absorption and utilization, potentially forming calcium oxalate when combined with calcium ions. Long-term excessive consumption may lead to kidney stones. Therefore, blanching spinach before consumption could be a wise choice. Despite its sour taste, lemon becomes alkaline after metabolism and is rich in vitamin C with powerful antioxidant properties. It stimulates the liver to produce digestive enzymes, aiding in breakdown and detoxification.

2. Apple + Celery + Carrot

This combination provides an abundance of antioxidants and essential nutrients, helping to accelerate detoxification and boost immunity. Apples, a common and nutrient-rich fruit, are alkaline and contain various vitamins, minerals, and antioxidants. They support digestion, strengthen immune function, and maintain the body's acid-base balance, promoting the detoxification process. Celery is high in dietary fiber, vitamin K, potassium, and small amounts of vitamin C, with properties that support diuresis, regulate blood pressure, and improve digestion.

3. Kale + Celery + Ginger + Lemon

Rich in a variety of vitamins, this combination enhances immunity, promotes metabolism, and supports detoxification. Kale is particularly abundant in vitamins K, A, and C, aiding liver detoxification and immune system support.

4. Kale + Spinach

Packed with chlorophyll and antioxidants, this blend helps eliminate free radicals, strengthen immunity, and support liver detoxification processes.

5. Lemon + Garlic + Turmeric + Black Pepper + Ginger + Olive Oil

When mixed thoroughly and left to rest in the refrigerator overnight, consuming 2-3 teaspoons daily can help reduce inflammation and eliminate toxins from the body. The combination of black pepper and turmeric, in particular, has potent anti-cancer properties, which are explored in detail in another section of this chapter.

6. Wheatgrass + Parsley + Lemon

This blend helps remove heavy metals, supports liver health, and enhances the body's detoxification capabilities. Wheatgrass is rich in chlorophyll, vitamins A, C, E, and iron, promoting liver detoxification.

7. Cucumber + Parsley + Ginger + Apple

This hydrating and diuretic combination helps maintain water balance in the body and promotes detoxification.

8. Celery + Lemon + Ginger

This blend aids digestion, promotes bowel movements, reduces inflammation, and supports liver detoxification.

The flexible combinations of these common vegetables, fruits, and flavorings provide comprehensive nutritional support in the short term, aiding detoxification and inflammation reduction while improving overall health.

Additionally, increasing the intake of raw vegetables in your daily diet, especially chlorophyll-rich green vegetables, can significantly enhance the body's detoxification functions by raising oxygen levels in the blood. A green vegetable salad is an excellent choice, as it is rich in vitamins, minerals, and antioxidants, promoting digestive health and supporting the body's natural detoxification process.

During the dandelion growing season, fresh dandelion leaves can be added to vegetable and fruit juices or salads. Since dandelion leaves may taste slightly bitter on their own, combining them with other ingredients improves palatability. This mix not only provides additional antioxidant support but also introduces potential anti-cancer nutrients into your diet. Active compounds in dandelions may inhibit cancer cell growth and boost immune function, helping to maintain a healthy balance in the body. Further exploration of dandelion's various benefits in the recovery process is covered later in this text.

In conclusion, whether for addressing current challenges or maintaining daily health, these ingredients offer sustained support and significant benefits, making them an ideal choice that should not be overlooked.

Selenium: A Key Trace Element For Detoxification

Excessive accumulation of toxins in the body can lead to various diseases. Therefore, when discussing dietary detoxification, selenium—a trace element essential for health—deserves special attention for its significant role in detoxification. Among the 15 essential trace elements, selenium is celebrated for its unique antioxidant and detoxifying properties, earning it the title of "nature's detoxifier" alongside chlorella. In China, selenium is referred to as the "king of anti-cancer," the "element of longevity," and the "guardian of health," underscoring its indispensability as a critical nutrient for life.

Key Benefits of Selenium for Human Health are as follows:

1. Detoxification, Protection Against Toxins, and Anti-Pollution

Selenium can bind to harmful metal ions such as mercury and lead, facilitating their elimination from the body. It also removes accumulated waste and toxins, reducing the toxic effects of chemical carcinogens, pesticide residues, and other pollutants. Consuming selenium-rich foods in appropriate amounts can effectively support detoxification and help the body resist environmental pollution.

2. Boosting Immune Function

Selenium plays a vital role in the immune system, enabling the identification of viruses, foreign substances, and diseased tissues within the body. It enhances the ability of immune cells to engulf pathogens, significantly strengthening the body's defense against diseases and building a robust barrier for overall health.

3. Prevention of Cardiovascular Diseases

Selenium provides powerful protection for the cardiovascular system and is often called the "guardian of the heart." Adequate selenium intake supports myocardial function, lowers the risk of atherosclerosis, and helps prevent coronary heart disease and hypertension.

4. Supporting Liver Health

As the body's primary detoxification organ, the liver plays a central role in metabolizing toxins and waste. Selenium enhances the liver's antioxidant capacity, accelerates the breakdown and metabolism of alcohol and other harmful substances, and helps repair liver cells, significantly reducing the risk of liver damage. For individuals who consume alcohol, appropriate selenium intake can effectively mitigate the harmful effects of alcohol on the liver. Additionally, selenium's detoxifying properties further contribute to liver health.

5. Antioxidant Effects and Delaying Aging

By activating key enzymes within the body's antioxidant system, selenium effectively inhibits the formation of free radicals and reduces oxidative damage to cells. This slows down aging and decreases the likelihood of chronic diseases. Studies have shown that individuals with higher blood selenium levels tend to live longer. Research by Chinese scientists has revealed that centenarians often have blood selenium levels three to six times higher than those of the average population.

6. Protecting Vision

Selenium plays an important role in maintaining eye health, improving vision, and preventing eye disorders. Long-term selenium deficiency can lead to vision decline and increase the risk of conditions such as cataracts.

7. Cancer Prevention and Anti-Cancer Effects

Research indicates a strong correlation between selenium intake levels and cancer risk. Chronic selenium deficiency increases the likelihood of cancer, while sufficient selenium intake can reduce cancer incidence by inhibiting cancer cell proliferation, inducing apoptosis in cancer cells, and alleviating oxidative stress. As a key component of antioxidant enzymes such as glutathione peroxidase, selenium neutralizes free radicals, protecting cells from oxidative damage and reducing the risk of cellular transformation into cancer cells. Additionally, selenium can alleviate the side effects of chemotherapy and radiation therapy, offering supportive protection for individuals undergoing cancer treatment.

In summary, selenium's potent antioxidant properties effectively inhibit the formation and spread of cancer cells, making it a critical element in cancer prevention.

Sources of Selenium and Dietary Considerations

Since selenium cannot be synthesized by the body, it must be obtained through daily dietary intake. Selenium-rich foods include Brazil nuts, seafood, poultry, grains, and eggs, with Brazil nuts being one of the best natural sources. However, due to their high selenium content, it is recommended to consume no more than two Brazil nuts per day.

The selenium content in different foods is significantly influenced by the selenium levels in the soil, as plants absorb selenium through their roots, and animals obtain selenium by consuming these plants or their derivatives. Therefore, the selenium content of the same type of plant or animal product can vary depending on its place of origin. For example, grains and vegetables grown in selenium-rich soil generally contain higher selenium levels than those from selenium-deficient areas.

A balanced and reasonable diet can effectively meet the body's daily selenium requirements, supporting immune function, antioxidant activity, and other vital physiological processes. This not only improves quality of life but also provides a foundation for long-term health and longevity. However, as selenium has a low requirement and a narrow safety margin, excessive intake can lead to health problems. Therefore, moderate and diversified consumption of selenium-containing foods is particularly important.

Selenium Supplements

Selenium supplements may be beneficial for individuals with additional needs, such as those who are selenium-deficient or have specific health concerns. It is essential to strictly control the dosage to avoid adverse effects from overconsumption. Consulting a healthcare professional before taking selenium supplements is recommended to determine the appropriate dosage and form. For healthy individuals, a balanced diet is typically sufficient to meet the body's daily selenium requirements.

Water: The Elixir Of Life

Water is a fundamental element of life, and adequate hydration is essential for everyone, especially for individuals whose health is more vulnerable, such as those affected by cancer. Maintaining proper hydration is particularly critical during the recovery process, as the body's demand for water increases. Water plays a vital role in regulating body temperature, supporting blood circulation, aiding digestion, transporting nutrients, eliminating waste, keeping the skin hydrated, and maintaining brain health.

Key Roles of Hydration During This Period are as follows:

1. Balancing Blood Sugar and Electrolytes
Adequate water intake helps regulate blood sugar and maintain electrolyte balance, which is especially important for individuals undergoing chemotherapy. Proper hydration supports stable blood sugar levels and balances electrolytes such as sodium, potassium,

and calcium, alleviating discomforts such as fatigue, dizziness, and muscle cramps, thereby reducing physical stress during this period.

2. Regulating Body Temperature and Tolerance

Body temperature regulation is crucial for comfort during cancer management. Sufficient hydration helps the body dissipate heat and maintain a balanced temperature. For individuals sensitive to temperature changes, staying well-hydrated can improve adaptability to fluctuations and alleviate discomfort caused by external temperature variations.

3. Supporting Kidney Function and Detoxification

Water plays a central role in kidney function and the body's detoxification processes. Proper hydration enhances the kidneys' ability to filter blood effectively, eliminating metabolic waste and preventing toxin buildup. This reduces the burden on both the liver and kidneys, promoting overall health. For therapies introduced later in this chapter—such as baking soda therapy—adequate hydration is especially important. It ensures optimal kidney function, preventing damage from excessive metabolic strain and supporting overall health. Additionally, water is vital in natural remedies discussed later, such as detox therapies, graviola leaf tea, and dandelion tea, where it serves as a key element.

4. Easing Discomfort and Supporting Inflammatory Balance

Adequate water intake supports normal metabolism and helps maintain a healthy inflammatory response, reducing the discomfort caused by excessive inflammation in tissues. Dehydration can increase physical stress, causing generalized or localized discomfort that affects the overall recovery experience. Maintaining hydration creates favorable conditions for the body to better manage the challenges of recovery, improving comfort throughout the healing process.

5. Promoting Wound Healing and Tissue Repair

For individuals undergoing surgery or invasive treatments, wound healing and tissue repair are paramount. Adequate hydration supports cellular metabolism and tissue regeneration, providing optimal conditions for wound healing. Proper hydration also positively impacts immune function, creating a supportive environment for the recovery process.

6. Maintaining Digestive Health and Nutrient Absorption

Water acts as a lubricant and softener in the digestive process, helping food and waste pass smoothly through the intestines and alleviating constipation and gastrointestinal discomfort. Common side effects during chemotherapy, such as dry mouth, constipation, and nausea, can be mitigated with proper hydration. Water softens stool, aids in effective nutrient absorption, and supports the digestive system's stability.

Additionally, the effectiveness of certain natural remedies, such as the combination of turmeric and black pepper discussed later, depends on a well-functioning digestive system. Proper hydration promotes the absorption and utilization of these components. Water not only delivers nutrients to cells but also fosters overall health and enhances the body's self-healing capabilities. Therefore, maintaining adequate hydration is foundational for digestion, nutrient absorption, and overall recovery.

7. Enhancing Immune Function and Lymphatic Drainage

Water is critical for the normal operation of the immune and lymphatic systems. Proper hydration ensures the fluidity of lymph, enabling white blood cells and immune cells to travel efficiently throughout the body, enhancing immune defense and toxin removal. Furthermore, during therapies such as mini-trampoline exercises for lymphatic drainage, discussed later in this text, adequate hydration is indispensable to ensure the lymphatic system's optimal function and further support detoxification.

8. Reducing Fatigue and Enhancing Stamina

Adequate hydration helps maintain normal blood flow, ensuring efficient oxygen and nutrient transport, which can alleviate fatigue during recovery. Proper water intake provides a solid foundation, helping individuals adapt better to the healing process.

9. Supporting Mental Health and Emotional Stability

Water positively impacts brain function and emotional regulation. Studies have shown that staying hydrated improves focus, reduces anxiety and fatigue, and promotes emotional balance, helping to alleviate the psychological stress associated with recovery.

The above highlights the critical support that proper hydration provides during the recovery process. Maintaining a scientific and reasonable hydration routine is particularly important. It is essential to avoid waiting until feeling thirsty to drink water; instead, water should be replenished regularly and systematically. Daily water intake should be adjusted based on individual health conditions, recovery plans, and daily habits, ensuring that the body consistently maintains optimal hydration levels.

In natural therapies, water plays an irreplaceable role in supporting the body's healing processes. It serves as a foundational measure for self-repair, contributing to enhanced overall recovery outcomes. Rehydrating the body is not limited to drinking water alone. Foods rich in water content—such as lettuce, tomatoes, cucumbers, zucchini, strawberries, citrus fruits, and coconut water—are excellent sources of hydration. Among these, cucumbers are particularly beneficial as they are high in water content and contain small amounts of vitamin K, which help maintain hydration and support kidney function. Their alkalizing properties promote effective hydration while enhancing urinary output, thereby assisting in cleansing the kidneys and eliminating bodily waste, further aiding detoxification.

These foods not only provide hydration but also supply essential vitamins and minerals to meet nutritional needs during recovery. Unsweetened herbal teas and homemade diluted fruit juices are also ideal hydration options, especially for those who may not prefer plain water. While these alternatives effectively contribute to hydration, they should not replace water as the primary source of fluid intake but rather complement it. Sugary or caffeinated beverages should be avoided, as excessive caffeine can have a diuretic effect, and sugary drinks may burden the kidneys, hindering detoxification and recovery.

During this time, I have developed the habit of drinking a glass of water before bed to ensure that the kidneys and liver can function more effectively during sleep. Proper hydration allows these organs to optimize their detoxification and metabolic processes. This effectiveness can often be observed in the color of morning urine. For those who wake during the night, consider stopping water intake at least one hour before bed to minimize nighttime interruptions and preserve sleep quality.

The above practices represent detoxification strategies I have adopted during recovery. A comprehensive application of these methods can support the body's natural detoxification processes, helping to eliminate harmful substances, strengthen the immune system, and enhance overall recovery. Incorporating these key factors into daily life not only aids recovery but also establishes a solid foundation for maintaining the body's pH balance.

In the following section on pH balance, we will explore various methods to help the body maintain this balance more effectively,

thereby promoting overall health and recovery.

Breathing And Holistic Balance: A Key To Health And Detoxification

Breathing is not only the force that sustains life but also a gateway to health. As a fundamental life function, it is a natural and unconscious process. However, mastering proper breathing techniques and practicing them intentionally holds immense value for both cancer recovery and overall health. As a simple yet effective method of health support, breathing exercises can significantly enhance immune function, optimize lung capacity, promote blood circulation, and effectively reduce stress and inflammation in the body. Moreover, an adequate oxygen supply is critical for maintaining the body's acid-base balance. Insufficient oxygen or an accumulation of carbon dioxide can lead to the formation of an acidic environment, disrupting normal metabolic processes, weakening the immune system, and affecting the body's recovery.

Key Benefits of Breathing Exercises are as follows:

1. Oxygen Supply and Cellular Metabolism

Proper breathing increases the body's oxygen supply, improving blood circulation and enabling cells to perform their metabolic functions more efficiently. Higher blood oxygen levels enhance the immune system's ability to fight infections, particularly by supporting lymphatic circulation, which aids in the removal of waste from the body. Oxygen, as a critical element of cellular metabolism, boosts cell vitality, supports tissue repair, and accelerates energy production.

2. Supporting Lymphatic Detoxification

Breathing stimulates and promotes the circulation of the lymphatic system, which helps remove toxins and waste from cells and tissues. The lymphatic system is a crucial mechanism for detoxifying the body, yet unlike the circulatory system, it lacks a "pump" to facilitate movement. The expansion and contraction of the thoracic cavity during breathing create pressure changes that drive lymphatic flow, aiding in the elimination of cellular and tissue waste.

3. Facilitating the Removal of Carbon Dioxide and Waste

Breathing is the primary mechanism for expelling carbon dioxide, a byproduct of cellular metabolism, from the body. While breathing itself does not directly eliminate toxins, it improves oxygen circulation and supports the removal of metabolic waste. Through breathing exercises, the efficient expulsion of carbon dioxide and other gaseous waste can be enhanced, reducing the body's acidic burden and promoting a healthy internal environment.

4. Stress Reduction and Hormonal Balance

Studies have shown that proper breathing provides significant benefits for stress management and mental health, particularly for individuals experiencing anxiety or depression. Breathing exercises increase oxygen supply to the brain, stabilize emotions, and activate the parasympathetic nervous system, thereby reducing the secretion of stress hormones such as cortisol.

From the above, it is evident that breathing is vital for overall health, and correct breathing practices offer numerous benefits. To begin breathing exercises, choose a quiet, well-ventilated environment. Relax your body, maintain a comfortable sitting or standing posture, and keep your back straight; some exercises can also be performed while lying down. By focusing on your breath, you can clearly feel the flow of air within your body, reflecting traditional Chinese medicine's emphasis on the movement of energy. Each individual may experience breathing exercises differently, and the benefits will vary from person to person.

Here are four common and easy-to-practice breathing exercises that can support overall health and detoxification:

1. Deep Abdominal Breathing

This technique involves slow and deep inhalations and exhalations designed to deliver more oxygen to the lungs. Abdominal breathing also relaxes the nervous system, alleviates stress, and effectively promotes lymphatic flow, indirectly enhancing the body's ability to fight infections and eliminate waste, thus supporting the immune system.

How to Practice:

Sit or lie down comfortably, placing both hands on your abdomen. Inhale deeply through your nose, allowing your abdomen—not your chest—to expand. Then exhale slowly through your mouth, feeling your abdomen gently deflate. Practice for about 5 minutes at a time, several times a day.

2. 4-7-8 Breathing Technique

The 4-7-8 breathing technique is a relaxation method that regulates the duration of inhalation, breath-holding, and exhalation. It is highly effective in reducing anxiety. This technique activates the parasympathetic nervous system, placing the body in a relaxed state and indirectly supporting detoxification. It balances oxygen and carbon dioxide levels, relieves stress, and promotes overall health.

How to Practice:

Inhale deeply through your nose for 4 seconds, hold your breath for 7 seconds, and then exhale slowly and completely through your mouth over 8 seconds. Repeat this cycle 4 to 5 times, practicing twice daily.

3. Alternate Nostril Breathing

This technique involves breathing alternately through each nostril, which helps balance brain function, increase oxygen intake in the lungs, relieve stress, and promote relaxation. Alternate nostril breathing also improves carbon dioxide elimination, supporting the body's natural detoxification processes.

How to Practice:

Using your right thumb, gently close your right nostril and inhale slowly through your left nostril. Then, use your right ring finger to close your left nostril, release your right nostril, and exhale slowly through the right nostril. Inhale again through the right nostril, then close it with your thumb and release your left nostril to exhale through the left side. Repeat this alternating pattern for about 5 minutes. Keep your breathing smooth and steady while remaining relaxed.

4. Walking with Deep Breathing

Combining deep breathing with walking in natural environments, particularly forests or areas with abundant greenery, can effectively boost metabolism, accelerate waste elimination, increase oxygen intake, improve blood circulation, reduce stress, and enhance overall health. During recovery, this practice supports the immune system and promotes the body's self-healing processes.

How to Practice:

Walk for 20 to 30 minutes in a natural setting while practicing deep breathing. Inhale deeply through your nose and exhale slowly through your mouth, maintaining a steady rhythm throughout the walk.

Incorporating Breathing Exercises into Daily Life

These exercises can be practiced flexibly according to individual needs, offering substantial benefits to the body. Regular practice of these techniques not only improves focus but also fosters a more positive mindset, balances the nervous system and hormone secretion, and enhances the body's self-healing and detoxification capabilities.

As discussed in Chapter 1, traditional Chinese medicine emphasizes that the root causes of illness often involve dampness, toxins, and stagnation of energy—issues such as poor circulation and toxin accumulation. Techniques like deep breathing and meditation are widely applied to promote mind-body balance and support the body's detoxification and prevention mechanisms.

While breathing exercises do not directly detoxify the body like the liver and kidneys, they indirectly contribute to self-cleaning and recovery by alleviating stress, boosting immunity, improving blood circulation, and enhancing sleep quality. This makes them a powerful complementary approach to optimizing overall health and supporting recovery.

Although not a direct cancer treatment method, these exercises strengthen the body's resilience to illness to some extent. Proper breathing not only improves physical health but also regulates mental and emotional states. Deep, steady breathing often reflects a state of inner peace, joy, and optimal well-being. Ancient Chinese wisdom suggests that human lifespan is linked to the number of breaths taken, emphasizing that slow and rhythmic breathing can clear the mind, stabilize emotions, and promote longevity.

It is evident that changing how we breathe can change the trajectory of our lives. Alongside dietary adjustments, quality sleep, and breathing exercises, stress management and mental health are also core elements of successful detoxification and recovery. In Chapter 6, we will further explore this topic and discuss strategies to comprehensively support the body's self-healing processes.

The Gut: A Core Force For Comprehensive Detoxification And Immunity

Gut health is essential for individuals of all ages. Known as the "second brain," the gut contains a vast network of nerve cells capable of processing information independently of the brain. This unique capability allows the gut to play a pivotal role not only in digestion and immune regulation but also in influencing emotions and overall well-being.

The gut is responsible for more than just digestion and nutrient absorption; it also helps lighten the body's toxic load by eliminating metabolic waste and toxins, thereby promoting overall recovery. When the gut functions optimally, detoxification processes become more efficient, contributing to enhanced systemic health.

Specifically, the role of the gut in maintaining health is reflected in the following aspects:

1. Waste Elimination

Smooth and regular bowel movements are critical for detoxification, effectively removing metabolic waste and harmful substances while preventing toxin accumulation. Consistent intestinal peristalsis is vital for maintaining the gut's detoxification function and supporting recovery.

2. Balancing Harmful Bacteria and Clearing Toxins

Beneficial gut bacteria help inhibit the growth of harmful bacteria, break down toxins, and reduce the burden of harmful substances from food. This process promotes nutrient absorption and maintains overall gut balance.

3. Supporting the Immune System

A healthy gut prevents harmful substances from entering the bloodstream and aids the immune system in defending against external threats and inflammation. It also fosters a balanced microbiota, which supports recovery and enhances overall health.

4. Preventing Toxin Reabsorption

A healthy intestinal mucosal barrier prevents toxins from re-entering the bloodstream and being reabsorbed by the body, thus avoiding secondary damage. Maintaining gut health effectively reduces the body's detoxification burden.

5. Assisting Liver Detoxification

The liver excretes certain toxins into the gut via bile, and a healthy gut ensures the efficient elimination of these toxins, reducing the liver's workload. By supporting gut detoxification, the gut also contributes to systemic metabolic balance, which can indirectly improve sleep quality and aid recovery.

As mentioned in the opening section of the detoxification chapter, the gut and sleep share a closely interdependent relationship. A balanced gut microbiota and quality sleep complement each other, playing a decisive role in overall health.

Adequate sleep is crucial for maintaining gut microbiota balance, protecting the intestinal barrier, and supporting detoxification processes. Sleep deprivation can lead to a reduction in beneficial bacteria and an increase in harmful bacteria, disrupting the diversity and stability of the microbiota. Chronic lack of sleep can also compromise gut barrier function, increase intestinal permeability (often referred to as "leaky gut"), and trigger systemic inflammation.

A healthy gut not only reduces inflammation, regulates emotions, and strengthens the immune system but also promotes better sleep quality. At the same time, sufficient sleep supports the repair of the intestinal mucosa and the maintenance of the gut barrier, further fostering microbiota balance and gut health. These two elements work synergistically, jointly regulating the immune system and ensuring the body operates at its best.

In summary, the intricate relationship between gut health and sleep quality underscores their cooperative roles in overall health. Together, they regulate and enhance immunity, detoxification, and recovery across multiple bodily systems, making them indispensable for achieving optimal well-being.

To sustain gut health and facilitate the body's recovery process, consider the following key aspects:

1. Foods to Avoid

Prolonged consumption of overly cold or spicy foods may irritate the stomach and intestines, leading to digestive discomfort. Opt for warm, easily digestible foods to reduce the burden on the digestive system and support gut health. Additionally, it is important to limit the intake of sugar and processed foods. High-sugar and heavily processed foods can disrupt the balance of gut microbiota and impair digestive function. Prioritize natural, whole foods to alleviate strain on the gut.

2. Regular and Balanced Eating Habits

A balanced diet is crucial for maintaining gut health. Avoid eating dinner too late; aim to finish your last meal at least four hours before bedtime, allowing the digestive system to rest overnight. A nutrient-rich, consistent eating routine ensures that the body absorbs essential nutrients and maintains the gut's normal functions.

3. Maintaining a Positive Mindset

The gut microbiota can influence emotional regulation. Maintaining a positive outlook helps balance hormone levels and reduces stress on the gut, thereby supporting overall health. Emotional fluctuations and gut discomfort are interconnected; the state of the gut often affects emotions and vice versa, highlighting the close relationship between the gut and mental well-being.

4. Adequate Hydration

Proper hydration promotes regular bowel movements, prevents constipation, and ensures smooth digestion. Tailor your daily water intake to your individual needs to support the gut's normal operations. Drinking warm water is gentler on the stomach and suitable for regular consumption. Additionally, the dietary strategies mentioned earlier can provide supplemental hydration as needed.

5. Moderate Exercise

Engaging in moderate physical activity can stimulate intestinal motility, help food move smoothly through the digestive tract, and prevent constipation, thereby improving gut health. Light exercises such as walking and yoga not only aid digestion but also relieve stress, making them excellent choices for maintaining gut well-being.

6. Abdominal Massage

If your physical condition allows, gently massaging the abdomen can be beneficial. Warm your hands by rubbing them together before massaging to enhance the effect and align the hand's temperature with the body. A common technique involves circular, clockwise motions around the navel, which align with the natural direction of intestinal peristalsis, thereby promoting digestion and detoxification.

According to traditional Chinese medicine, the abdomen is considered the "seat of the spleen and stomach," a vital area for the flow of qi (energy. and bodily fluids. Regular abdominal massage can enhance spleen and stomach function, relax the body, and improve gut and overall health. For optimal results, perform abdominal massages upon waking, before bed, or about 30 minutes after meals. This practice can effectively improve blood circulation, stimulate meridians, harmonize qi and blood, and enhance gastrointestinal muscle tone, accelerating intestinal motility and supporting digestion and nutrient absorption.

Abdominal massage is also helpful for alleviating bloating and constipation while promoting gut health. Pairing massage with deep breathing can further relax the body and amplify the benefits. However, outcomes vary by individual, so adjust massage techniques and pressure according to personal needs to ensure suitability.

7. Avoid Overuse of Antibiotics

Antibiotics should only be used when necessary, as they not only eliminate harmful bacteria but can also disrupt the beneficial bacteria in the gut, affecting overall gut health. Overuse of antibiotics may lead to microbial imbalances, increasing the risk of infections and other health issues. During antibiotic use, consider taking probiotics to help maintain a balanced microbiota and mitigate the negative effects of antibiotics on the gut. Antibiotics should always be used under medical supervision to protect gut function as much as possible.

When discussing gut health, fermented foods such as sauerkraut are an indispensable nutritional choice and a valuable addition to a gut-friendly diet. Research has shown that sauerkraut promotes detoxification, regulates the body's acid-base balance, and provides significant benefits for gut health. These findings have been validated by scientific studies. Incorporating sauerkraut into your daily diet not only improves digestive function but also plays a critical role in maintaining overall health and balance.

The Mechanisms Behind Sauerkraut's Health Benefits are as follows:

1. Supporting Digestion and Detoxification

Sauerkraut is rich in lactic acid bacteria, which studies have shown to improve the diversity and balance of gut microbiota, enhancing digestive health and immune system functionality. The probiotics produced during fermentation help maintain a healthy gut microbiome, thereby promoting digestion. Additionally, the dietary fiber and enzymes in sauerkraut aid in clearing intestinal toxins, assisting the body in its natural detoxification processes.

2. Regulating Acid-Base Balance

While sauerkraut has a tangy, acidic taste, its metabolism in the body produces an alkaline effect, helping to maintain the body's acid-base balance. Research indicates that foods with an alkaline metabolic effect can reduce the body's acid load, contributing to a healthier pH equilibrium.

3. Strengthening the Immune System

The probiotics and antioxidants in sauerkraut, such as vitamin C, are beneficial for boosting immunity. These components enhance the body's resistance to toxins and reduce the risks associated with inflammation and toxin accumulation. The critical role of vitamin C and probiotics in supporting immune health has been extensively studied, demonstrating their antioxidative and anti-inflammatory effects.

Although sauerkraut offers certain benefits for digestion and acid-base balance, it serves as a supplementary measure rather than a primary solution for overall health management. For optimal results, sauerkraut should be combined with other health strategies.

In addition to these benefits, stress management and minimizing exposure to harmful substances play essential roles in supporting gut health. Together, these factors ensure the smooth operation of the gut's functions in digestion, nutrient absorption, and detoxification, maintaining a positive cycle that further stabilizes mood and the immune system.

The human body possesses innate self-cleansing and detoxification mechanisms, primarily relying on the liver, kidneys, intestines, and skin. The primary goal of detoxification is to enable more efficient nutrient absorption, which can typically be supported through healthy lifestyle habits without the need for detox products or extreme detox regimens, as such methods may have adverse effects on the body.

Maintaining gut health and overall bodily balance requires the synergistic effect of multiple factors. When the body's systems function optimally, toxin accumulation is minimized, reducing the burden on organs like the liver and kidneys. This also improves nutrient absorption efficiency, ensuring that vital nutrients are effectively delivered to cells throughout the body, thereby supporting overall health.

The digestive system is intricately linked to the gut, with the gut playing a critical role in food breakdown, nutrient absorption, and waste elimination. Gut health directly impacts the overall functionality of the digestive system, including nutrient absorption efficiency and the body's detoxification capabilities. When gut function is compromised, it can lead to malnutrition, weakened immunity, and even broader digestive system issues.

In summary, gut health is essential for the body's recovery and overall well-being. The juicing therapies introduced in this section, combined with the alkaline dietary approaches in the following section, along with healthy lifestyle practices such as quality sleep and moderate exercise, create a synergistic effect. Together, these measures optimize detoxification, support gut health, and promote holistic health.

pH Balance: The Foundation of Health

In the previous discussion on water, the concept of pH was briefly introduced. The acid-base balance within the body is critical for maintaining normal metabolic and physiological functions. Blood pH typically remains within a narrow range of 7.35 to 7.45, which is slightly alkaline. This balance is vital for the proper functioning of enzymes, efficient oxygen transport, and the stability of cellular metabolism. Any significant deviation from this range can have adverse effects on health.

To maintain this acid-base equilibrium, the body relies on the coordinated efforts of the respiratory system, kidney function, and internal buffering systems. These mechanisms work together to regulate blood pH strictly, ensuring the body can adapt to external environmental changes and metabolic activity fluctuations, thereby sustaining overall physiological balance and health.

In contrast, urine pH is more variable, typically ranging from 4.5 to 8. It serves as an indirect indicator of the body's acid-base balance. In healthy individuals, urine pH usually falls between slightly acidic and neutral (6.0 to 7.5).

In many cases, individuals with cancer may experience a slightly more acidic bodily fluid environment. This is often due to acidic byproducts, such as lactic acid, produced by the metabolic activity of cancer cells in localized areas. A basic understanding of the body's acid-base status can be obtained by measuring urine pH. Urine pH provides some clues about the body's overall acid-base balance and serves as an initial reference. pH test strips, which are widely available at most pharmacies, offer a convenient method for this assessment.

Timing and Considerations for Measurement

The ideal time to measure urine pH is the first urine of the morning, as it reflects the body's metabolic state after a night of rest. Morning urine is generally less influenced by external factors, offering a more accurate representation of kidney acid excretion and the body's overall acid-base balance.

However, it is important to note that a single measurement cannot comprehensively reflect the body's acid-base status. Only by conducting multiple measurements and tracking trends over time can one gain a more reliable and accurate understanding of the body's pH balance.

The Impact of Diet and Exercise on Urine pH

Certain dietary choices and physical activities can significantly influence urine pH. Consuming alkaline-rich foods tends to increase urine pH, while high-protein diets can lead to a decrease. Additionally, intense physical exercise, particularly anaerobic activities such as sprinting or strength training, can result in the production of lactic acid. This lactic acid buildup temporarily lowers both blood and urine pH, causing a slight acidity. Such changes are short-lived, and as the body recovers and clears lactic acid, pH levels gradually return to normal. Therefore, to obtain more accurate and stable results, it is generally not recommended to measure urine pH immediately after meals or intense exercise.

During cancer recovery, avoiding strenuous exercise is equally important. Excessive physical exertion can place additional stress on the body, potentially compromising immune function and slowing recovery progress. Gentle, restorative forms of exercise, such as light stretching or walking, are more beneficial for recovery. Most importantly, the intensity of exercise should be adjusted according to individual physical conditions to ensure both safety and effective rehabilitation.

Dynamic Nature of Urine pH

Urine pH is dynamic and influenced by multiple factors beyond diet and exercise, including metabolic state and medication use. Therefore, careful attention should be given to the timing and frequency of testing to ensure more accurate and meaningful results. Regular monitoring and recording of urine pH trends, in conjunction with an overall assessment of health, can provide better insights into the body's acid-base balance.

If there are any concerns, it may be helpful to consult a medical professional. Maintaining a proper acid-base balance plays an important role in overall health. Through appropriate dietary adjustments and healthy lifestyle habits, it is possible to effectively support the body's pH balance, creating an environment less conducive to cancer cell growth and fostering overall health improvement.

In summary, maintaining the body's acid-base balance can be achieved through a combination of internal and external strategies. Detailed step-by-step guidance on specific approaches and methods will be provided in the following sections to help you better understand and apply these techniques.

Alkaline Diet: Supporting Cancer Recovery And Overall Health

Scientific research has demonstrated that a balanced diet not only significantly promotes recovery by providing essential nutrients but also plays a critical role, particularly when centered around plant-based foods rich in antioxidants and fiber.

The detoxifying fruit and vegetable juices mentioned earlier are an excellent example, as they are packed with a variety of antioxidants and protective nutrients that effectively enhance the body's ability to combat oxidative damage. These juices not only aid in detoxification but also protect cells from free radical damage, boost the body's self-repair mechanisms, and support the immune system, making them more effective in inhibiting the growth of cancer cells. As such, they form an integral part of an alkaline diet.

In addition to the cancer-fighting fruits and vegetables previously discussed, many other alkaline foods can help regulate the body's pH levels, creating a more favorable alkaline internal environment to support cancer recovery.

Top Alkaline Foods Known for Their Health Benefits are as follows:

1. Leafy Greens

Examples: spinach, arugula, lettuce, malabar spinach, mustard greens, cilantro, and celery (cilantro can be used as both a herb and a vegetable).

These vegetables are rich in chlorophyll and minerals such as magnesium and potassium. As mentioned earlier, spinach is notable for its cleansing properties, which help remove heavy metals and other toxins from the body. Leafy greens also help regulate the body's pH levels and reduce inflammation, making them an indispensable component of an alkaline diet.

2. Cruciferous Vegetables

Examples: broccoli, kale, cabbage, and cauliflower.

Cruciferous vegetables are packed with vitamin C, fiber, and antioxidants. They contain glucosinolates, which are converted during digestion into isothiocyanates, the most notable being sulforaphane. Sulforaphane exhibits anti-inflammatory, antioxidative, and detoxifying properties and has demonstrated anti-cancer potential in experimental studies.

Broccoli sprouts, in particular, have gained attention for their exceptional anti-cancer properties. Research by Dr. Paul Talalay and his team at Johns Hopkins University found that broccoli sprouts contain 10 to 100 times the concentration of glucoraphanin compared to mature broccoli. Sulforaphane inhibits cancer cell growth through various mechanisms, including neutralizing free radicals, reducing inflammation, inducing apoptosis in cancer cells, and inhibiting tumor angiogenesis. Daily consumption of a small amount of broccoli sprouts is considered a simple yet effective anti-cancer dietary choice.

3. Beets

Beets are rich in betaine and pectin, which provide powerful detoxifying effects and support liver health. They help purify the blood, stimulate bile production, and aid digestion and detoxification. The antioxidants in beets improve blood circulation, further enhancing the body's natural detoxification processes.

4. Citrus Fruits

Examples: lemons, oranges, and grapefruits.

Citrus fruits are abundant in vitamin C and antioxidants, which help neutralize free radicals in the body. Lemon juice, in particular, stimulates digestion, supports liver function, and aids in detoxification.

5. Dark-Colored Berries

Examples: blackberries and blueberries, as well as other multi-enzyme fruits.

These berries are rich in health-promoting nutrients, including anthocyanins, vitamins, minerals, and dietary fiber. These components make dark-colored berries powerful antioxidants that protect the body from free radical damage, reducing oxidative stress on cells. Additionally, these berries support gut health and promote the proper functioning of the digestive system. The anthocyanins not only give these berries their deep purple or blue hues but also play a significant role in anti-inflammatory and anti-cancer processes.

6. Avocado

Avocado is a nutrient-dense superfood rich in glutathione, a potent antioxidant that neutralizes acidic substances in the body and supports liver detoxification. Avocados also provide healthy fats, particularly monounsaturated fatty acids, which improve the absorption of fat-soluble vitamins such as vitamins A, D, E, and K. These vitamins, along with the fiber content in avocados, promote cardiovascular health and digestive system function. The antioxidants in avocados also help eliminate free radicals in the body, further enhancing liver detoxification.

7. Legumes and Nuts

Legumes are rich in fiber, which aids digestion and helps reduce cancer risk. Nuts contain omega-3 fatty acids known for their anti-inflammatory properties. Additionally, the vitamin E and selenium in nuts offer powerful antioxidant benefits, protecting cell membranes and promoting overall health. Almonds, in particular, are among the few nuts with alkaline properties. They are high in calcium and magnesium, which support bone health and help maintain the body's acid-base balance.

8. Apple Cider Vinegar

Apple cider vinegar has gained popularity for its numerous health benefits. It is rich in vitamins, minerals, organic acids, and antioxidants, supporting digestion, boosting immunity, balancing blood sugar levels, improving skin health, and regulating the body's pH levels. As a natural food product, apple cider vinegar promotes liver function and aids in the elimination of waste, making it an excellent choice for daily health and detoxification.

Research suggests that consuming apple cider vinegar in moderation or incorporating it into meals can support cardiovascular health and assist with weight management, thereby contributing to overall wellness.

Apple cider vinegar can be used in salad dressings, marinades, or cooked dishes, adding a unique flavor and acting as a natural preservative. It can also be prepared as a beverage by mixing 1 to 2 tablespoons of apple cider vinegar with 200 to 250 milliliters of drinking water. Stir well and enjoy. This simple method is both convenient and health-promoting. Consuming 1 to 2 servings per day, with 1 to 2 tablespoons per serving, is sufficient. For those who dislike plain water, this serves as a flavorful alternative.

To protect dental health, consider rinsing your mouth after drinking apple cider vinegar to minimize potential damage to teeth. Individuals with sensitive stomachs should wait at least 30 minutes after meals before consuming it to avoid excessive irritation, as drinking it on an empty stomach may negatively impact the gastric mucosa.

9. Chlorella and Kelp

As discussed earlier in this chapter on detoxification, chlorella and kelp are notable for their unique detoxifying properties. Additionally, they are considered alkaline foods that help balance the body's pH levels and reduce the impact of acidic diets.

Modern dietary patterns often include large quantities of acidic foods, such as meat, processed foods, and sugar, which can increase the body's acid burden. Reducing the intake of such foods while incorporating mineral-rich alkaline foods like chlorella and kelp can support pH balance and indirectly promote overall health.

10. Green Tea

Green tea is rich in catechins, which support liver function and aid in detoxification. It also boosts metabolism and assists in fat burning. In the following sections, additional teas with unique supportive roles in cancer prevention will be discussed.

To better support an alkaline balance, it can be beneficial to moderate the consumption of acidic foods such as red meat, sugar, processed foods, alcohol, and coffee, as these may affect the body's acid-base equilibrium. The impact of meat and sugar on cancer prevention will be further explored in subsequent content.

In summary, choosing alkaline foods provides essential nutritional support and sustained energy during the cancer recovery process. Increasing the intake of alkaline-rich foods helps effectively regulate the body's pH levels, laying a solid foundation for overcoming disease and promoting overall health.

Baking Soda: Supporting Ph Balance And Aiding Recovery

The potential application of baking soda in cancer care primarily lies in its ability to regulate and neutralize acidity within the body. By lowering acidity levels and inhibiting fungal growth, baking soda may interfere with the rapid proliferation of cancer cells in acidic environments. Since cancer cells tend to thrive and spread more effectively in acidic conditions—as highlighted in previous discussions—alkalizing the body's internal environment may help inhibit further expansion of cancer cells.

Usage Instructions

A common method involves mixing one teaspoon of baking soda with two tablespoons of maple syrup, heating the mixture until caramelized, and consuming it in divided doses. This approach is based on the theory that the sugar in maple syrup attracts cancer cells, while the alkaline properties of baking soda alter the acidic environment of these cells, disrupting their growth.

Another approach is preparing baking soda water. Dissolve one teaspoon of baking soda in 300 ml of drinking water, stir well, and consume. For optimal effectiveness, it may be helpful to drink this solution after dinner, once digestion is mostly complete, to reduce any potential interference with stomach acid. In other words, consuming it on an empty stomach is ideal. This not only helps maintain hydration levels during the night but also supports kidney detoxification and efficiently regulates the body's pH balance.

To continuously monitor the body's pH levels, regular use of pH test strips is recommended. Ensuring the pH remains within an optimal range may contribute to the body's self-healing capabilities and provide additional health benefits.

Precautions

While baking soda has garnered attention in certain alternative therapies, its usage requires caution. The dosage of orally consumed baking soda should be strictly controlled, as excessive intake may result in side effects such as metabolic alkalosis or gastrointestinal discomfort. Therefore, it is essential to use it in moderation and carefully observe the body's response to ensure both safety and efficacy.

It is particularly important to emphasize that baking soda should be considered part of a comprehensive recovery plan rather than a standalone therapy. As an auxiliary measure, it should be combined with other restorative approaches to ensure compatibility and overall effectiveness while minimizing potential risks.

Alkaline Bath: Regulating Ph And Supporting Detoxification

An alkaline bath is a holistic immersion therapy often used as a complementary practice. By adding baking soda and salt to bathwater to raise its pH level to an alkaline state (typically above 7), this therapy aims to balance the skin's pH, while also soothing the body and mind, relieving stress, and improving skin health. Additionally, it has a positive effect on the normal functioning of the immune system.

From the perspective of Traditional Chinese Medicine (TCM), alkaline baths offer several supportive benefits:

1. Regulating Yin-Yang Balance

TCM places great importance on maintaining yin-yang balance. Alkaline baths help relax the body and mind by adjusting the skin's pH environment, particularly during recovery periods. As a supportive measure, it aids in achieving a harmonious state, complementing other treatments and interventions.

2. Promoting Qi and Blood Circulation

TCM identifies poor circulation of qi and blood as a significant cause of illness. The warmth provided by an alkaline bath relaxes muscles and enhances circulation, helping to alleviate blockages that may arise during the recovery process. This, in turn, strengthens the body's natural self-healing capacity.

3. Eliminating Dampness and Toxins

According to TCM, cancer is often linked to the accumulation of toxins in the body. Alkaline baths open the pores, facilitating the removal of dampness and toxins and boosting the skin's metabolic functions. This indirectly supports detoxification and strengthens the body's resistance against cancer.

4. Calming Emotions and Spirit

TCM emphasizes emotional well-being, as imbalances in emotions can lead to stagnation of qi and blood, potentially triggering or worsening illness. The relaxing effects of an alkaline bath help reduce anxiety and tension, calming the mind and mitigating the impact of negative emotions on health.

Usage Instructions

Alkaline baths can be performed regularly based on individual needs while being thoughtfully adjusted to one's physical condition, especially for individuals with weak immunity or overall poor health. In the initial stages, starting with higher water temperatures and longer soaking times can be beneficial, provided they align with personal comfort levels.

As the body gradually adapts, the duration of the bath can be extended to 20–30 minutes to maximize its benefits, effectively aiding in the regulation of the body's pH balance. The ideal time for an alkaline bath is at least one hour after a meal to avoid disrupting digestion. After the bath, it is recommended to hydrate adequately to maintain fluid balance and support metabolism.

In summary, an alkaline bath is a simple and gentle complementary therapy that supports the body's natural detoxification processes, balances pH levels, alleviates stress, and promotes overall health recovery. When practiced moderately and consistently, alkaline baths help maintain the balance of qi and blood within the body, sustain vitality during recovery, and provide effective support for holistic well-being.

Silica: A Source Of Cellular Health

Silica is a naturally occurring mineral and an essential trace element with numerous health benefits. It plays a meaningful role in natural cancer therapies by supporting the health of skin, hair, nails, connective tissues, and bones, while also exhibiting anti-inflammatory properties and promoting cellular regeneration. These functions indirectly enhance the immune system. By fortifying cellular structures and aiding detoxification processes within the body, silica contributes to improved overall health and offers valuable support for cancer defense.

Dietary Sources of Silica

Silica can be incorporated into the diet through natural sources such as whole grains, legumes, and drinking water. These sources typically provide adequate amounts to meet the body's needs for this trace element. For those with specific health conditions requiring additional supplementation, maintaining appropriate dosage levels is important to avoid long-term or excessive intake. When prolonged use is considered, it can be beneficial to seek guidance from a healthcare professional to ensure safe and effective usage.

Applications of Silica

1. Topical Use

Silica is often applied externally in gels or creams to support skin care. These products contribute to skin repair, promote faster healing, and improve overall skin health.

2. Oral Use

Silica is available in liquid or powder forms as a dietary supplement, aiding cellular health and enhancing immune function. Regular intake, such as two tablespoons per day, may help maintain an alkaline environment in the body and inhibit the growth of cancer cells.

In summary, incorporating silica into daily routines, whether through diet or supplementation, supports overall health while offering vital protection throughout the process. By bolstering the body's natural defenses and strengthening cellular integrity, silica proves to be a reliable ally in promoting well-being and addressing health challenges.

Detoxification and pH Balance: A Synergistic Relationship

In the previous sections, we explored specific methods for detoxification and pH regulation in the body. These two processes are closely intertwined, complementing each other in maintaining health. Detoxification, as a critical step in removing harmful substances and metabolic waste from the body, not only optimizes bodily functions but also effectively contributes to pH balance. Conversely, achieving an ideal pH state helps sustain the acid-base equilibrium post-detoxification, further promoting healing and overall health. This comprehensive approach—eliminating internal obstacles through detoxification and fortifying health by regulating pH—represents a scientific and holistic health management strategy.

The Interconnection Between Detoxification and pH Balance is as follows:

1. Detoxification's Impact on pH Balance

During detoxification, the body removes accumulated toxins and waste, many of which can increase acidity within the system. For instance, the buildup of metabolic waste can create an acidic environment. By eliminating these acidifying substances, detoxification helps the body more easily maintain or restore a healthy pH balance.

2. pH Balance's Role in Supporting Detoxification

Maintaining a proper acid-base balance enhances the function of vital detoxification organs such as the liver and kidneys. An overly acidic internal environment can impair the metabolic efficiency of these organs, reducing their detoxification capacity. Therefore, dietary and lifestyle practices that regulate pH levels effectively support the body's detoxification functions.

3. Enzymatic Activity and Metabolism

The body's acid-base balance (pH level) directly influences the activity of enzymes and metabolic processes. Enzymes generally function optimally within a specific pH range. Maintaining a balanced pH ensures the proper function of metabolic processes, including those involving detoxification enzymes. These enzymes play a crucial role in the liver and other organs, breaking down and expelling toxins from the body.

4. Liver Function

As the primary detoxification organ, the liver requires a suitable pH environment to efficiently process and eliminate harmful substances. An imbalanced pH, particularly one that skews acidic, can disrupt liver function and compromise detoxification capabilities.

5. Kidney Function

The kidneys eliminate acidic waste and other toxins through urine while also regulating the body's pH levels. They function most effectively within a stable pH environment, ensuring efficient waste removal. Maintaining acid-base balance is therefore essential for supporting the kidneys' detoxification role.

6. Inflammation and Toxin Accumulation

An acidic internal environment can promote inflammation, which in turn exacerbates the accumulation of toxins. By regulating pH levels and reducing acidity, inflammation can be minimized, indirectly aiding detoxification processes.

In summary, detoxification and pH regulation work synergistically in health management, providing mutual support during the recovery process. By promoting the body's natural detoxification mechanisms and maintaining acid-base balance, this dual strategy optimizes the internal environment, enhancing overall health. Together, they support the body's self-healing processes, laying a solid foundation for comprehensive health management and recovery while fostering lasting improvements in well-being.

The Synergistic Effect of Natural Ingredients: The Potential Benefits of Combinations

In addition to the nutrient-rich foods previously introduced, common kitchen spices also exhibit remarkable anti-cancer potential. Research has shown that these ingredients not only enhance the immune system but also effectively inhibit cancer cell growth through various mechanisms. Among these, the golden combination of turmeric and black pepper, as well as the powerful trio of onions, ginger, and garlic, stand out as exemplary. These spices are also seamlessly incorporated into the aforementioned fruit and vegetable juice blends.

Next, we will delve into how these potent ingredients provide robust support in the fight against cancer and explore their unique advantages in promoting overall health.

Turmeric And Black Pepper: A Potent Golden Duo

In our earlier discussion of detoxifying fruit and vegetable juices, we mentioned a combination that includes turmeric and black pepper. Here, we provide a detailed explanation of the anti-cancer properties of this pairing and the scientific evidence supporting it.

Turmeric is renowned for its anti-inflammatory, antioxidant, and potential anti-cancer properties. It supports liver function and aids digestion and detoxification by stimulating bile secretion. However, the primary active component of turmeric—curcumin—has extremely low bioavailability. This means that after ingestion, curcumin is poorly absorbed by the body and is quickly metabolized and excreted, limiting its effectiveness.

The active compound in black pepper, piperine, significantly enhances the absorption of curcumin. Piperine increases intestinal permeability and inhibits liver enzymes responsible for breaking down curcumin, prolonging its retention in the body. This synergistic effect maximizes the health benefits of curcumin, particularly its potential anti-cancer effects. The combined use of turmeric and black pepper is demonstrably more effective than using turmeric alone.

Multiple studies have confirmed that piperine can increase the bioavailability of curcumin by up to 20-fold. As previously noted, piperine inhibits specific enzyme systems in the liver, reducing curcumin metabolism and extending its duration in the body. This significantly enhances curcumin absorption and utilization. This discovery, originally published in a 1998 study in Planta Medica, has since been widely validated in subsequent research, highlighting the numerous health benefits of this combination. The conclusion is now well-recognized in nutrition science and natural medicine.

Therefore, when aiming to optimize turmeric's health benefits, pairing it with black pepper is essential to enhance curcumin absorption. Additionally, since curcumin is fat-soluble, combining it with fatty foods such as coconut oil, butter, or other oils can further promote its absorption. Higher concentrations of curcumin are particularly effective in reducing inflammation, combating oxidative stress, and inhibiting cancer cell growth.

Another convenient option is to use ready-made turmeric and black pepper capsules. These capsules not only significantly improve turmeric absorption but also offer unparalleled convenience. Portable and easy to take, they are especially suitable for integrating into a busy anti-cancer routine, allowing individuals to effortlessly reap the combined health benefits of these two powerful ingredients.

Onions, Ginger, And Garlic: Natural Anti-Cancer Powerhouses

Onions, ginger, and garlic are indispensable health-promoting ingredients in daily diets, celebrated for their anti-inflammatory and antioxidant properties. These foods are widely recognized for their potential to inhibit cancer cell growth, and regular consumption may help reduce the risk of various cancers.

Onions

Onions are rich in quercetin, a powerful antioxidant that neutralizes free radicals and reduces oxidative stress. This compound may play a key role in inhibiting cancer cell growth.

Ginger

Ginger, included in the detox juice combinations discussed earlier, is packed with active compounds such as gingerols and shogaols. These compounds exhibit strong anti-inflammatory and antioxidant properties, support digestive health, alleviate nausea, promote liver function, and improve blood circulation, enabling the body to more effectively eliminate toxins. Its anti-inflammatory effects also help mitigate inflammation-related health issues, offering overall protection and enhancing well-being.

Heating ginger enhances its health benefits by activating and releasing its active components, making them more bioavailable. For example, heated ginger releases higher concentrations of compounds like zingerone, which amplifies its anti-inflammatory, antioxidant, digestive, and immune-boosting effects. Moderate heating improves ginger's impact on digestive and circulatory health, making its benefits even more pronounced.

Garlic

Garlic is known for its potent antibacterial properties, which are most effective when consumed raw. To maximize its health and anti-cancer benefits, garlic can be chopped and left to sit for about 10 minutes before consumption. This process allows the release of allicin, a compound with significant antimicrobial and anti-cancer effects.

In summary, the sulfur compounds, aromatic hydrocarbons, vitamins, minerals, and fiber in onions, ginger, and garlic support normal metabolic functions and overall health. Notably, these ingredients regulate immune system function, helping the body fight diseases more effectively.

While onions, ginger, and garlic have promising anti-cancer properties, excessive intake may cause digestive discomfort. Moderate consumption tailored to individual tolerance optimizes their role in complementary therapies. Research also suggests that these ingredients can enhance the effectiveness of chemotherapy, boost the efficacy of anti-tumor drugs, and reduce the side effects of treatment.

To fully benefit from their health-promoting properties, these ingredients should be regularly incorporated into the diet, preferably raw or lightly cooked to retain their active compounds.

Supportive Measures: Cutting Off Cancer Cells' Energy Supply

In the fight against cancer, dietary adjustments play a crucial role in promoting recovery, as previously mentioned. Specifically, making targeted modifications to certain food choices not only helps maintain nutritional balance but also effectively weakens the "energy supply" of cancer cells, creating more favorable conditions for recovery. Below, we will explore the scientific basis behind several dietary strategies and their pivotal role in the anti-cancer process.

In addition to the dietary strategies discussed earlier, here are other adjustments I implemented during this process:

Adjusting Dietary Choices: Reducing Milk And Meat Consumption To Aid Recovery

Excessive intake of high-protein diets derived from meat and dairy products can generate acidic byproducts during metabolism, such as urea, which may lower urinary pH and create an acidic internal environment. To address this, protein requirements can be met through plant-based sources, which, when appropriately combined with diverse ingredients, ensure comprehensive nutritional support.

Moderate consumption of high-quality animal proteins, such as fish, eggs, and poultry (white meat), can provide the body with essential nutrients. In particular, fish rich in omega-3 fatty acids offer notable anti-inflammatory benefits, making them especially advantageous in this context. High-quality proteins enhance immune function, maintain muscle mass, and support physical strength. When consumed in moderation, these animal proteins complement plant-based dietary principles by ensuring adequate protein intake, aiding recovery, and promoting overall health and accelerated healing.

The key considerations regarding milk and meat during recovery are as follows:

1. Increased Inflammatory Response

Inflammation is closely linked to cancer progression, particularly in individuals with lactose intolerance or milk protein allergies. Some studies suggest that dairy products and red meat may exacerbate inflammation, potentially creating favorable conditions for tumor growth.

2. Insulin-like Growth Factor-1 (IGF-1)

Milk contains IGF-1, an insulin-like growth factor that promotes cell growth and division. Research indicates that elevated levels of IGF-1 may be associated with an increased risk of certain cancers. Reducing milk consumption could help lower the associated cancer risks.

3. Animal Fats

Red meat, especially processed varieties, is high in saturated fats and has been linked to an increased risk of cancer. During recovery, reducing or avoiding such foods may lower potential risks and support the overall healing process.

4. Acid-Base Balance

Milk and meat are classified as acidic foods. As noted earlier, excessive consumption can foster an environment conducive to cancer cell growth. Based on this premise, many natural therapies advocate for a reduced intake of acidic foods to help maintain the body's acid-base balance and enhance its self-repair mechanisms.

5. Nutritional Alternatives

Reducing the intake of milk and meat while increasing plant-based foods can significantly elevate dietary levels of fiber, antioxidants, and phytonutrients. These components strengthen the immune system, reduce inflammation, and support the body's natural detoxification processes.

By incorporating these adjustments, individuals can optimize their dietary choices to better support recovery, enhance overall well-being, and create a more balanced internal environment conducive to healing.

To better facilitate rapid recovery, consider incorporating the following plant-based protein sources into the diet, ensuring sufficient protein intake:

1. Legumes

Examples include lentils, chickpeas, black beans, and red beans.

2. Soy Products

Options like tofu, soy milk, and fermented soy products.

3. Nuts and Seeds

Such as almonds, walnuts, pumpkin seeds, flaxseeds, and chia seeds.

4. Whole Grain

Including quinoa, brown rice, and others.

These foods are not only rich in protein but also provide essential nutrients. However, certain plant-based foods may lack one or more essential amino acids. For instance, legumes are often low in methionine, while grains typically have limited lysine content. Therefore, plant proteins are sometimes referred to as "incomplete proteins" because they do not provide a balanced proportion of all essential amino acids required by the body.

By combining different plant-based protein sources, their amino acid profiles can complement each other to form a "complete" protein.

For example:

1. Pairing legumes with whole grains.

2. Combining nuts and seeds with legumes or grains.

These combinations create amino acid synergy, meeting the body's requirements for essential amino acids.

Plant-based foods are rich in antioxidants, dietary fiber, and phytochemicals. These components help neutralize free radicals, reduce oxidative stress, and possess anti-inflammatory properties. Additionally, they promote healthy gut motility, support gut health, and balance the gut microbiome. A healthy gut microbiome is crucial for a properly functioning immune system, which is scientifically recognized as essential in preventing the spread of cancer cells, particularly during cancer recovery.

In summary, dietary adjustments should be tailored to individual needs during recovery to ensure sufficient intake of proteins, vitamins, and minerals, thereby maintaining internal balance. A well-rounded nutritional structure provides critical support for the body's recovery and overall health.

Reducing Traditional Table Salt: Opting For Healthier Alternatives

Reducing the intake of traditional refined table salt is a dietary adjustment worth considering during special health periods. Compared to regular table salt, natural sea salt and Himalayan salt undergo less processing and retain more natural minerals, such as calcium, magnesium, potassium, and iron. These trace elements help maintain electrolyte balance, support metabolism, and contribute positively to overall health.

Refined table salt typically loses some of its minerals during processing. In contrast, the natural components found in sea salt and Himalayan salt are more aligned with the body's nutritional needs. These salts not only satisfy the salty flavor required in daily meals but also provide additional nutritional support.

When choosing salts, it may be beneficial to consider these natural alternatives while taking into account individual health conditions, dietary preferences, and nutritional requirements. Rich in a variety of minerals and trace elements, they offer essential nutritional benefits, supporting overall well-being and laying the foundation for optimal bodily functions.

Avoiding Refined Sugar: Blocking Unhealthy Energy Sources

Sugar is an irresistible temptation for many, but it also serves as a primary energy source for cancer cells during their metabolic processes. Research indicates that cancer cells preferentially utilize glucose through the "Warburg Effect," meaning they consume sugar at a much higher rate than normal cells. While sugar itself does not directly cause cancer, a high-sugar diet may indirectly facilitate cancer cell proliferation by increasing insulin and insulin-like growth factor 1 (IGF-1) levels.

High-sugar diets can lead to chronic inflammation and metabolic syndrome, creating an environment conducive to cancer cell growth. By managing blood sugar levels and reducing insulin production, it is possible to inhibit tumor progression to some extent. Low-carbohydrate, low-sugar diets reduce glucose availability in the bloodstream, limiting the energy source for cancer cells and supporting the recovery process.

Studies suggest that low-sugar diets may help slow the progression of cancer. Reducing the intake of refined sugar is critical for maintaining stable blood sugar levels, as refined sugar causes rapid spikes in blood sugar, providing "fuel" for cancer cells and promoting their growth. For individuals who find it challenging to eliminate sugar completely, natural sugar sources or alternatives can be used as transitional tools to help the body adapt gradually.

Additionally, reducing sugar intake incrementally, combined with appropriate psychological support and dietary adjustments, can ease the mental and physical discomfort associated with sugar withdrawal. Rather than abruptly cutting out sugar, a gradual reduction allows the body to adapt to new dietary habits, minimizing mood swings and energy dips during the transition. Treating the avoidance of refined sugar as a supportive recovery measure can help alter the metabolic environment of cancer cells and aid in the healing process.

Opting for nutrient-rich alternatives not only satisfies taste preferences but also provides beneficial micronutrients to support overall health. This gradual improvement approach not only reduces the negative health impacts of sugar but also fosters the development of long-term healthy eating habits.

When avoiding refined sugars, the following natural sugar sources can serve as healthier alternatives:

1. High-Quality Honey

Rich in antioxidants and small amounts of vitamins and minerals, honey can offer additional health benefits. However, it should still be consumed in moderation to avoid excessive sugar intake.

2. Fructose

Naturally found in fruits, fructose provides some vitamins and fiber. Compared to pure fructose, the fructose in whole fruits is absorbed more slowly due to their high fiber content, reducing its direct impact on blood sugar levels.

3. Maple Syrup

With a lower glycemic index (GI) than refined sugars, maple syrup contains beneficial minerals like manganese and zinc. Nonetheless, it should also be consumed in moderation.

4. Coconut Sugar

Containing small amounts of fiber, such as inulin, coconut sugar has a relatively low glycemic index and releases energy gradually, making it gentler on blood sugar levels.

5. Stevia

A zero-calorie plant-based sweetener, stevia does not cause blood sugar spikes, making it an excellent choice for those looking to reduce sugar intake or manage blood sugar levels.

Precautions for Natural Sugar Consumption

Although these alternatives are relatively healthier and help minimize sharp blood sugar fluctuations, they should be consumed in moderation according to individual health conditions and nutritional needs. Excessive reliance on any single sugar source should also be avoided. Fructose, in particular, is metabolized primarily in the liver, and excessive intake may lead to risks such as non-alcoholic fatty liver disease, insulin resistance, and elevated blood lipid levels. This could increase the likelihood of obesity, type 2 diabetes, and cardiovascular diseases.

Consuming whole fruits typically does not lead to excessive fructose intake because the dietary fiber and other nutrients in fruits help slow down the digestion and absorption of fructose, resulting in a more stable impact on blood sugar levels. However, it is important to consume fruits with high sugar content in moderation to avoid excessive sugar intake. Overall, opting for low-sugar fruits is more beneficial for blood sugar management. Additionally, as it is generally uncommon to consume an excessive number of fruits within a short period, eating whole fruits usually does not cause significant blood sugar fluctuations.

Traditional Chinese Medicine Perspective

In traditional Chinese medicine (TCM), most fruits are considered to have a "cooling" nature, particularly those with high water content or a sweet or sour taste. TCM suggests that overconsumption of cooling foods may harm the spleen and stomach's "yang energy," increasing the digestive system's burden and disrupting the balance of "qi and blood." Therefore, TCM advises moderate fruit consumption, especially for individuals with a "cold constitution" or weak spleen and stomach, to avoid exacerbating the body's cooling tendencies.

In summary, in special health periods, if refined sugar intake cannot be entirely avoided, choosing healthier natural sugar alternatives can support overall well-being and help maintain stable blood sugar levels. This approach not only benefits health management but also helps balance the immune system, contributing to overall health. Dietary adjustments play a crucial role in supporting recovery, and managing sugar intake is a strategy worth adopting.

The Power of Nature: Anti-Cancer Foods

During my battle against cancer, I incorporated two natural foods into my diet, both widely recognized for their remarkable anti-cancer potential. Research has shown that these foods not only effectively inhibit the growth of cancer cells but also enhance the body's self-repair capabilities.

In the following, we will explore how these two foods, through their unique active components, can effectively support the fight against cancer :

Bitter Almonds: The Potential Of Natural Remedies

Bitter almonds are a commonly known food containing amygdalin, also referred to as vitamin B17. This compound releases cyanide when metabolized in the body, which is theorized to have toxic effects on cancer cells. As such, amygdalin has garnered attention in some alternative medicine circles for its potential to suppress cancer cells, particularly within the realms of traditional and alternative therapies.

However, it is essential to note that cyanide is toxic not only to cancer cells but also poses potential risks to normal cells. Excessive consumption may lead to cyanide poisoning, posing significant health hazards.

Specific Benefits of Bitter Almonds as a Natural Remedy

1. Digestive System Support

In certain traditional medicine practices, bitter almonds have been used to promote digestive health. Their natural bitterness can stimulate the secretion of digestive fluids, supporting normal intestinal function.

2. Antioxidant Properties

Bitter almonds contain various antioxidants that neutralize free radicals, potentially protecting cellular health. These antioxidant properties suggest potential applications in overall health support and anti-aging.

3. Anti-Inflammatory Effects

Components of bitter almonds have demonstrated anti-inflammatory properties in some studies, which may help alleviate inflammation-related health issues. These properties are also thought to have a regulatory effect on the immune system.

4. Respiratory Health

In traditional pharmacology, bitter almonds have been used to help relieve coughs and bronchial problems. Their components are believed to have a soothing effect on the respiratory tract.

Guidelines for Safe Consumption

To minimize potential risks, it may be a good idea to gradually increase the intake of bitter almonds. Start with three almonds per day, evenly distributed throughout the day, and increase by one almond daily until reaching a maximum of 18 almonds per day. Do not exceed this limit. If adverse reactions occur, cease further increases immediately. Additionally, avoid consuming bitter almonds simultaneously with Salvestrol capsules; further details on Salvestrol will be provided below.

Important Considerations

It is crucial to emphasize that bitter almonds should only be used as a supplementary measure within a comprehensive therapeutic plan, rather than as a sole treatment. Close monitoring of the body's response is essential to prevent potential adverse side effects or toxic reactions. Particular caution should be exercised with raw bitter almonds, and they should only be consumed under appropriate guidance.

Grape Seed Powder: Exceptional Anti-Cancer Properties

Grape seed powder, made by drying and grinding grape seeds into a fine powder, is highly regarded for its potent antioxidants, such as proanthocyanidins. Particularly in cancer prevention and recovery, it has demonstrated remarkable potential. These antioxidants help neutralize free radicals, reduce oxidative stress, protect cells from damage, and may effectively inhibit cancer cell growth through their anti-inflammatory and antioxidant properties.

Key Benefits of Grape Seed Powder in Cancer Recovery

1. Rich in Proanthocyanidins

Proanthocyanidins, powerful antioxidants found in grape seed powder, enhance vascular health by relaxing smooth muscles in blood vessel walls, improving elasticity, and promoting better blood flow. These properties help prevent arteriosclerosis, regulate blood pressure, and support heart health.

2. Anti-Inflammatory Properties

Grape seed powder exhibits strong anti-inflammatory effects, reducing chronic inflammation in blood vessels and surrounding tissues. Since inflammation is closely associated with cancer development and progression, reducing inflammatory responses can help inhibit the growth and spread of cancer cells.

3. Antioxidant Action

The antioxidants in grape seeds neutralize free radicals, reduce oxidative stress, and protect against inflammation. Oxidative stress is a major factor in vascular endothelial damage and DNA damage. By protecting blood vessel walls and maintaining elasticity, antioxidants may lower cancer risk and improve circulatory function.

4. Dual Support for Vascular Health and Microcirculation

The oligomeric proanthocyanidins (OPCs) in grape seed extract are instrumental in promoting vascular health and improving blood circulation. They expand blood vessels, enhance their elasticity and strength, and reduce the risk of blockages, arteriosclerosis, and thrombosis. Research also shows that grape seed extract strengthens capillaries and microvessel walls, which is crucial for ensuring effective oxygen and nutrient delivery to tissues through healthy microcirculation.

5. Enhanced Immune Function

Nutrients in grape seed powder boost the immune system's ability to combat cancer cells and other harmful cells, thereby supporting overall health.

6. Promoting Cancer Cell Apoptosis

Studies suggest that proanthocyanidins in grape seed powder may induce apoptosis (programmed cell death) in cancer cells. This mechanism triggers the self-destruction of cancer cells, slowing tumor progression.

7. Inhibiting Tumor Growth

Antioxidants in grape seed extract have shown positive effects in inhibiting the proliferation of tumor cells in certain cancers, such as skin, breast, and prostate cancers, helping slow cancer progression.

Here are some reasonable ways to consume grape seed powder:

1. Mixing with Beverages

Stir grape seed powder into warm water or juice for a nutritious drink.

2. Adding to Foods

Incorporate grape seed powder into salads, soups, or dressings to enhance nutritional value. It can also be added to baked goods to increase dietary fiber and other nutrients but should be used under low-temperature conditions to preserve its active components.

3. Pairing with Other Nutrients

Combine grape seed powder with foods rich in vitamin C (e.g., citrus fruits, kiwis, red peppers, and strawberries) or those containing vitamin E and coenzyme Q10. While fat-soluble antioxidants primarily protect cell membranes, the water-soluble antioxidants in grape seed powder neutralize free radicals outside cells. These combinations create a synergistic effect that maximizes nutritional benefits.

Using these methods, you can effectively integrate grape seed powder into your daily diet. A recommended daily intake is 1 to 2 teaspoons, which can be adjusted based on individual needs to ensure safe and appropriate consumption.

In summary, with its potent antioxidant, anti-inflammatory, and cancer cell-inhibiting properties, grape seed powder serves as a valuable supportive tool in the recovery process. It enhances the body's resistance and promotes overall health improvement, making it a beneficial addition to a comprehensive health regimen.

Nutritional Supplements: Pillars of Health and Immunity

Under normal circumstances, a balanced and well-rounded diet can meet the nutritional needs of a healthy individual. However, for individuals with cancer, particularly those in advanced stages, nutritional supplements may become a critical and timely source of support. Illness often impairs the body's ability to absorb nutrients, making it challenging to fulfill dietary needs through food alone in the short term. In such cases, appropriate nutritional supplements can rapidly deliver essential nutrients, bolster the immune system, maintain energy levels, and support overall recovery. Thus, nutritional supplements serve as a valuable complement to regular diets in special circumstances, enhancing recovery outcomes and improving quality of life.

On my journey to overcome cancer, nutritional supplements became an indispensable part of my recovery. This was due to the following challenges I faced:

1. Urgency of Time

At that time, my health was critically fragile. Weighing under 50 kilograms despite a height of nearly 1.85 meters, I was severely weakened by the toll of cancer. While I tried to obtain nutrients through regular meals, I also needed to rapidly replenish my body with adequate nutrition and energy to regain strength and restore basic vitality within a short period.

2. Increased Nutritional Demands

For individuals affected by cancer, the body often requires additional specific nutrients to support immune function, antioxidant activity, and cellular repair. These heightened nutritional needs are difficult to meet through diet alone. Nutritional supplements became a vital resource for me, effectively supporting my immune system and helping to fend off further disease progression. They accelerated improvements in my nutritional status, provided me with precious recovery time, and became an irreplaceable part of my support system.

3. Absorption Efficiency

In certain cases, cancer or the recovery process can affect the digestive system, reducing the body's ability to efficiently absorb nutrients from food. Supplements can provide concentrated doses of essential nutrients in forms that are easier for the body to absorb and utilize, thereby meeting critical nutritional needs.

4. Loss of Appetite

Like many others affected by cancer, I experienced a significant loss of appetite, making it difficult to obtain sufficient nutrition through regular meals. Nutritional supplements served as a more convenient and effective alternative, helping to maintain my body's nutritional balance during this challenging time.

In summary, Nutritional supplements can be a crucial tool during recovery, providing essential nutrients in a short time to help combat illness and promote healing. However, it is important to note that excessive intake of supplements may hinder recovery or even have adverse effects on the body. Moderation and balance are key to ensuring the best outcomes from supplements. When necessary, their use should be guided by a doctor or professional nutritionist to ensure safety and efficacy.

In addition to maintaining as normal a diet as possible, the following supplements provided me with essential additional nutritional support:

Salvestrol Capsules: A Natural Anti-Cancer Force

Salvestrols are phytonutrients found in certain fruits and vegetables that have gained attention in recent years for their potential anti-cancer properties. They are commonly used as supportive supplements in cancer recovery. The unique feature of Salvestrols is their ability to be metabolized by the CYP1B1 enzyme, which is selectively expressed in cancer cells, into toxic compounds that can destroy cancer cells while sparing healthy cells. Salvestrol capsules are available in concentrated and standardized doses, making them particularly suitable for individuals who may not obtain sufficient Salvestrols through their regular diet.

Purchasing and Usage Guidelines

Salvestrol capsules can be purchased from regulated pharmacies or legitimate online platforms. Choosing certified suppliers is a critical step in ensuring product quality.

When using Salvestrol capsules, especially in conjunction with other supplements or medications, certain precautions are necessary. For example, some components in bitter almonds may interfere with the metabolic pathway of Salvestrols, affecting the activity of the CYP1B1 enzyme and thereby reducing their anti-cancer effectiveness. To avoid potential efficacy reduction or adverse reactions, it is important to allow a time interval between consuming bitter almonds and taking Salvestrol capsules, ensuring that both can exert their optimal anti-cancer effects.

Important Considerations

While Salvestrols are considered to have anti-cancer potential, they should be used as a supportive measure in conjunction with other health strategies rather than as a standalone therapy. Combining them with a holistic approach ensures the most effective support for cancer recovery.

Liquid Zinc: Core Support For The Immune System

Zinc is one of the essential trace elements required by the

human body, playing a vital role in enhancing immune response, promoting wound healing, and improving the body's ability to resist infections and diseases. During the battle against illness, zinc's significance becomes even more pronounced. Its anti-inflammatory properties help mitigate inflammatory responses within the body while protecting cells from oxidative stress. For individuals affected by cancer, sufficient zinc intake can provide critical support during recovery, aiding in overall health restoration.

The key functions of zinc are as follows:

1. Anti-Inflammatory Properties

Zinc has notable anti-inflammatory effects, inhibiting the production of certain inflammatory factors. This helps reduce chronic inflammation, thereby lowering the risk of cancer associated with inflammation.

2. Antioxidant Effects

As an effective antioxidant, zinc protects cells from oxidative damage caused by free radicals. By reducing oxidative stress, it helps lower the risk of cancer cell formation.

3. Immune System Support

Zinc is essential for the proper functioning of the immune system. Adequate zinc levels enhance the efficiency of immune cells in identifying and destroying cancer cells, strengthening the body's anti-cancer defenses.

4. DNA Repair

Zinc is a critical component of various DNA repair enzymes. It supports the repair of damaged DNA, reducing the risk of mutations. By aiding in the restoration of normal cell function, zinc lowers the probability of cancer development.

5. Inhibition of Cancer Cell Proliferation

Research indicates that zinc can influence the division and proliferation of cancer cells. By inhibiting specific signaling pathways and targeting key enzymes and proteins involved in cancer cell growth, zinc can effectively slow down or even stop the spread of cancer cells.

6. Promotion of Apoptosis

Zinc activates specific apoptotic pathways, triggering the self-destruction of abnormal cells. This reduces the number of cancer cells and inhibits tumor formation and expansion.

These diverse mechanisms make zinc a critical element in supporting the body and aiding in cancer prevention and management.

Zinc Intake Methods

1. Liquid Zinc Supplements

Liquid zinc supplements are often considered the most effective form of zinc intake due to their ability to be absorbed quickly and efficiently by the body. This makes them particularly suitable for individuals with weakened digestive systems or absorption challenges. Liquid zinc is available over the counter and can be easily purchased at pharmacies or online as part of a daily dietary supplement routine.

2. Natural Dietary Sources

Zinc can also be obtained through a balanced diet. Foods rich in zinc include meat, fish, oysters, nuts, seeds, egg yolks, whole grains, and legumes. These natural food sources not only provide ample zinc but also contribute to overall health through diverse nutritional combinations.

Important Considerations

While zinc offers numerous health benefits, excessive intake may lead to side effects, such as gastrointestinal discomfort or interference with the absorption of other minerals. When using supplements, it is essential to adhere to the recommended dosage to ensure safety and effectiveness. However, consuming zinc through a normal diet rarely poses a risk of overconsumption. Properly managed, zinc intake is a valuable tool for supporting immune health, combating disease, and promoting recovery.

Vitamin C: A Powerful Anti-Cancer Booster

Vitamin C is an essential water-soluble vitamin for the human body. It functions as an antioxidant and a cofactor for various enzymes, playing a critical role in numerous physiological processes. Unlike most vertebrates, humans are unable to synthesize vitamin C due to genetic factors, making it necessary to obtain it through food or supplements.

Many individuals affected by cancer often have insufficient vitamin C intake, which can lead to weakened immunity and hinder the recovery process. Given my condition at the time, I began supplementing vitamin C in the early stages. In special circumstances, high-dose vitamin C administered under medical supervision can be considered to enhance its potential anti-cancer supportive effects.

The key benefits of Vitamin C are as follows:

1. Enhanced Antioxidant Action

Vitamin C is a powerful antioxidant that neutralizes free radicals, reducing oxidative stress and DNA damage. High doses of vitamin C can further amplify antioxidant defenses, helping to mitigate cell damage during the early stages of cancer and inhibit the spread of cancer cells.

2. Boosted Immune System Function

Vitamin C supports the immune system by activating immune cells such as macrophages and T cells. High-dose vitamin C enhances the body's immune response, aiding in the efficient identification and attack of cancer cells, thereby improving anti-cancer effectiveness.

3. Inhibition of Cancer Cell Proliferation

Studies have shown that high-dose vitamin C injections can selectively exhibit toxicity to cancer cells without harming normal cells. This occurs because high concentrations of vitamin C produce excessive hydrogen peroxide, which damages cancer cells and inhibits their growth and proliferation.

4. Improved Chemotherapy and Radiotherapy Outcomes

High-dose vitamin C injections may help alleviate common side effects of chemotherapy and radiotherapy, such as nausea, fatigue, and immunosuppression. Research suggests that vitamin C can have a synergistic effect, supporting the efficacy of these treatments while reducing their impact on healthy tissues.

5. Support for Collagen Production

Vitamin C is essential for collagen synthesis, aiding in the repair and protection of damaged tissues. Many affected individuals experience tissue damage, and high doses of vitamin C, by promoting collagen production, contribute to tissue repair and overall health recovery.

Important Considerations

Beyond its anti-cancer support, vitamin C may also improve appetite, reduce fatigue, alleviate depression, and enhance sleep quality. However, high-dose vitamin C injections should be viewed as a complementary therapy rather than a primary treatment method.

While vitamin C is critical for health, excessive intake is not recommended. According to the Chinese Nutrition Society, a daily intake of 200 milligrams is advised for chronic disease prevention. Overconsumption of vitamin C can lead to gastrointestinal discomfort, including nausea, vomiting, and acid reflux symptoms.

In summary, high-dose vitamin C injections may support early cancer recovery by enhancing immune function, reducing free radical damage, and mitigating treatment side effects. However, it is crucial to consult with a physician before using such therapies to assess individual health conditions and needs, ensuring their safety and appropriateness.

Vitamin D3: A Key Enhancer Of Immunity

In recent years, Vitamin D3 has gained significant attention in cancer research. Studies indicate that a deficiency in Vitamin D is closely linked to the development of various diseases, including weakened immune defenses, and may increase the risk of cancer. For individuals affected by cancer, maintaining adequate Vitamin D3 levels not only boosts immunity but also plays a critical role in calcium regulation and bone health.

This group often requires more Vitamin D3 than the general population due to the disease process, which can accelerate calcium loss and heighten the risk of osteoporosis. Vitamin D3 aids in calcium absorption in the intestines, improving the body's ability to utilize and store calcium, thereby maintaining strong and healthy bones. Additionally, Vitamin D3 helps regulate immune responses, assisting in the detection and elimination of cancer cells while promoting recovery. As such, it is widely recognized as an important supportive measure in cancer recovery and prevention.

By combining sunlight exposure, a balanced diet, and supplements when necessary, individuals can effectively raise their Vitamin D3 levels, ensuring optimal calcium utilization and enhancing the body's ability to manage the challenges of cancer recovery.

Key Benefits of Vitamin D3 in Cancer Recovery

1. Boosting the Immune System and Reducing Chronic Inflammation

Vitamin D3 regulates the immune system by activating immune cells, which play a crucial role in identifying and eliminating cancerous cells. Furthermore, its significant anti-inflammatory properties help reduce chronic inflammation in the body, inhibiting the onset and progression of cancer. This effect is particularly vital in preventing the spread of cancer cells and enhancing overall anti-cancer efficacy.

2. Regulating Cell Differentiation

Vitamin D3 is essential in regulating cell proliferation and differentiation, suppressing the growth of abnormal cells while promoting the healthy development of normal cells. By inducing apoptosis (programmed cell death), Vitamin D3 helps inhibit the spread and metastasis of cancer cells.

3. Inhibiting Tumor Angiogenesis

Vitamin D3 limits the formation of new blood vessels (angiogenesis) within tumors, reducing their ability to obtain nutrients and oxygen.

Since tumors rely on new blood vessel growth for sustenance, inhibiting angiogenesis helps slow their growth and spread.

4. Alleviating Depression

Cancer often imposes both physical and emotional stress, and Vitamin D3 may play a positive role in this regard. Depression is a common challenge during cancer treatment. By regulating the immune system and reducing inflammation, Vitamin D3 not only supports anti-cancer efforts but also helps alleviate depressive symptoms. Its dual role in addressing depression and cancer makes it a promising adjunctive therapy when combined with medical treatments and psychological support, ensuring both physical and mental well-being.

5. Synergistic Effects with Conventional Therapies

Vitamin D3 may complement traditional treatments such as chemotherapy and radiotherapy by supporting the recovery process. Research suggests that Vitamin D3 helps mitigate common side effects, such as fatigue and immunosuppression, enabling individuals to better endure these treatments and promoting overall recovery.

In summary, vitamin D3 plays a significant supportive role in cancer prevention and recovery, serving as a vital tool in enhancing immune function, managing health, and bolstering disease resistance. For both individuals affected by cancer and healthy populations, adequate Vitamin D3 intake is crucial to maintaining immunity and improving overall health outcomes.

The primary sources of vitamin D3 include its synthesis in the skin through sunlight exposure and certain foods rich in vitamin D. If necessary, vitamin D3 supplementation can be considered to address deficiencies and ensure adequate levels in the body.

Intake and Related Information About Vitamin D3

Synthesis Through Sunlight

The human body synthesizes Vitamin D3 when the skin is exposed to ultraviolet B (UVB) rays. Research indicates that UVB radiation is strongest around midday, making this time the most efficient for Vitamin D3 production in the skin. However, prolonged exposure to intense sunlight can damage the skin and increase the risk of premature aging. To avoid harmful effects, it may be wise to limit direct sun exposure between 10 a.m. and 2 p.m. during the summer months. Opting for early morning or late afternoon sunlight not only protects the skin but also optimizes Vitamin D3 synthesis.

Under suitable conditions, the skin can produce approximately 1,000 IU of Vitamin D3 per minute of sunlight exposure. A 10 to 30-minute exposure can generate 10,000 to 25,000 IU, which is typically sufficient to meet most individuals' daily Vitamin D requirements. The synthesized Vitamin D3 can be stored in the body for use during periods of limited sunlight. However, individual Vitamin D3 needs vary based on factors such as age, health status, and conditions of sun exposure. Efficiency of synthesis is also influenced by several factors, including skin tone, geographic location, season, obstacles blocking sunlight, and personal sensitivity to UV rays.

Modern lifestyles and work environments often limit sun exposure, particularly in winter or regions with limited sunlight, leading to a decline in Vitamin D levels in the body. With prolonged lack of sunlight, the body gradually depletes its stored Vitamin D3, reducing its ability to maintain adequate levels. As a result, incorporating dietary sources or supplements into one's routine has become an effective solution for maintaining healthy Vitamin D3 levels.

By addressing these challenges proactively, individuals can ensure adequate Vitamin D3 intake to support overall health and well-being.

Calcium Absorption and Vitamin D: Ideal Food Choices

In addition to the alkaline diet introduced in Section 3 of this chapter and the plant-based protein foods mentioned in Section 5, incorporating the following food categories can more effectively promote calcium absorption. Some of these foods also serve as excellent sources of vitamin D:

1. Sesame and Sesame Paste
These foods have a higher calcium content than vegetables and legumes.

2. Almonds
Among the nuts, almonds are one of the richest sources of calcium.

3. Dried Figs
Rich in calcium, magnesium, potassium, and vitamin K, dried figs contribute to bone health. Notably, magnesium supports calcium absorption.

4. Fatty Fish, Fish Roe, and Small Fish Bones
These foods are not only significant sources of calcium but are also rich in vitamin D, particularly in fatty fish varieties.

5. Eggs
Especially egg yolks, which are excellent sources of vitamin D.

6. Dried Mushrooms

Mushrooms, such as shiitake or white mushrooms, treated with sunlight or ultraviolet light, contain higher levels of vitamin D2 and aid calcium absorption.

7. Liver

Animal liver, such as beef or chicken liver, provides a moderate amount of vitamin D.

8. Dried Shrimp

These small, sun-dried shrimps are known as "natural calcium supplements" due to their exceptionally high calcium content, surpassing that of fish and eggs.

9. Seaweed (Nori)

As a member of the red algae family, seaweed is a nutrient-dense food found in marine environments. It is rich in protein, minerals, and dietary fiber, with calcium, magnesium, iron, and iodine being particularly abundant. Among vegetables and algae, seaweed stands out for its calcium content.

These foods play a vital role in supplementing vitamin D and enhancing calcium absorption, making them key dietary sources of this essential nutrient. Vitamin D2 (ergocalciferol) is predominantly found in plants and fungi, such as mushrooms and yeast, while vitamin D3 (cholecalciferol) is primarily derived from animal-based foods, including fish, liver, and egg yolks.

Both vitamin D2 and D3 play crucial roles in maintaining adequate vitamin D levels in the body, promoting calcium absorption and supporting bone health. However, they differ slightly in their absorption and metabolism. Research indicates that vitamin D3 remains in the body longer and is more effective at raising blood vitamin D levels. Consequently, D3 is generally considered more efficient in sustaining the body's vitamin D reserves.

While maintaining bone health is essential for daily life, it becomes even more critical in specific medical situations, particularly during cancer treatment. Chemotherapy and radiation therapy often result in bone loss or osteoporosis, significantly increasing the body's demand for nutrients and highlighting the importance of bone health. Maintaining a healthy bone marrow environment is vital for the proper functioning of the immune system, which plays a key role in combating cancer cells. Moreover, bone health is closely linked to overall nutrition. Adequate intake of calcium, vitamin D, magnesium, and other essential nutrients not only strengthens bones but also enhances immunity and promotes overall well-being.

A balanced diet and regular exercise can effectively slow down bone loss. Routine bone density monitoring helps assess bone health. A nutritious diet not only replenishes calcium but also ensures the intake of other essential nutrients such as iron, vitamin K, vitamin C, phosphorus, magnesium, potassium, and zinc. These nutrients work synergistically with vitamin D3 to enhance calcium metabolism and absorption, aid in bone repair, and support the body's normal functions.

In addition to proper nutrition, regular physical activity is critical for maintaining bone health. Weight-bearing exercises stimulate bone remodeling and formation, increasing bone density and strength. Gentle activities such as swimming, tai chi, and Baduanjin help improve joint flexibility and balance, slowing joint aging. Strong muscles also reduce stress on bones, further protecting bone and joint health.

The effective utilization of calcium relies on the combined actions of various nutrients, particularly magnesium, potassium, and vitamin K, which play key roles in bone health. Magnesium activates vitamin D, enhancing calcium absorption, while potassium reduces calcium loss through urine, helping to retain calcium in the bones. Thus, a nutrient-rich diet provides the essential elements needed for bone health and minimizes calcium depletion.

Vitamin D3 has a particularly close relationship with calcium. Adequate vitamin D3 supports the efficient absorption and storage of calcium, promotes the health of bones and teeth, and maintains calcium balance in the blood, ensuring the body's physiological functions operate smoothly.

Foods That Affect Calcium Absorption

To support optimal calcium absorption and utilization, it can be helpful to moderate the intake of high-salt, fried, high-fat foods, carbonated beverages, high-protein diets, strong tea, excessive coffee, excessive alcohol, sugary processed foods, and foods high in oxalates. These items can lead to calcium loss or hinder its absorption by various mechanisms, such as increasing calcium excretion or interfering with its metabolism and uptake. Notably, excessive smoking and alcohol consumption suppress the function of osteoblasts (bone-forming cells), increasing the risk of osteoporosis.

Excessive intake of sodium chloride in salt disrupts calcium metabolism. A high-salt diet promotes sodium excretion, and calcium is simultaneously lost through urine. Long-term consumption of excessive salt may lead to calcium depletion, negatively impacting bone health. Similarly, excessive alcohol reduces the activity of osteoblasts, raising the risk of osteoporosis. Fried and high-fat foods impair calcium absorption, while the phosphoric acid in carbonated beverages may interfere with calcium metabolism. High-protein diets accelerate calcium excretion. Furthermore, certain compounds in strong tea and excessive coffee inhibit calcium absorption.

Overall, a balanced diet is essential for promoting calcium absorption and utilization, playing a critical role in preventing osteoporosis. Maintaining dietary diversity and moderation while avoiding excessive consumption of the aforementioned foods supports healthy calcium absorption and bone health.

Guidance on Vitamin D Supplementation

If dietary intake of vitamin D is insufficient, vitamin D3 supplements can serve as a quick and effective short-term source to maintain healthy vitamin D levels in the body. While vitamin D3 is vital for health, excessive intake may lead to hypercalcemia, adversely affecting the kidneys, cardiovascular system, central nervous system, and even bones. It may also interfere with the absorption of other trace elements. Typically, determining the appropriate supplementation dose through blood tests to assess current vitamin D levels is the most effective approach.

Guidelines For Nutritional Supplements

For most healthy individuals, a balanced diet typically provides sufficient nutrients to meet daily needs without requiring additional supplements or health products. For those with special needs or who are unable to maintain a proper diet, high-quality supplements may serve as appropriate nutritional support when used under the guidance of healthcare professionals.

Professor Tim Spector, a genetic epidemiologist and nutrition scientist at King's College London, has warned about the potential health risks associated with nutritional supplements, particularly calcium supplements. He noted that individuals who take calcium tablets regularly over an extended period may face a higher risk of heart disease, as certain supplements can deposit in the arteries, potentially leading to arterial calcification over time. Consequently, he advocates obtaining nutrients primarily from natural food sources rather than relying on supplements, as some supplements may pose health risks.

Vitamins are generally categorized into two types:

1. Water-soluble vitamins (such as B vitamins and vitamin C): Excess amounts are typically excreted through urine.

2. Fat-soluble vitamins (such as vitamins A, D, E, and K): These can accumulate in the body, and excessive long-term intake may pose health risks.

The optimal approach is to work with a physician or dietitian to assess individual needs, ensuring supplement usage is appropriate to avoid deficiencies or overdoses while maximizing safety and effectiveness. Once the body achieves balance, the use of vitamin supplements should be carefully managed. A well-balanced diet is the preferred method for maintaining long-term and sustainable health.

Cancer-Fighting Herbs: The Healing Power of Nature

In my journey of combating cancer, alongside the aforementioned strategies, certain traditional herbs have demonstrated remarkable healing potential. In the section on alkaline diets earlier in this chapter, we discussed the unique anti-cancer properties of green tea. In this section, we will focus on two additional natural plants with notable cancer-fighting effects: Graviola leaf tea and dandelion. These plants are not only renowned for their ability to support the immune system and promote overall health but also exhibit significant potential in the fight against cancer.

We will now explore how these two herbs, through their distinct mechanisms of action, provide essential support in this process:

Graviola Leaf Tea: Support In Combating Cancer

Graviola, also known as soursop, is a tropical fruit renowned for its potential health benefits. As a traditional herbal tea, Graviola leaf tea has garnered attention for its antioxidant, anti-inflammatory, and immune-supporting properties, particularly in the context of recovery and complementary support. Made from the leaves, bark, or fruit of the Graviola plant, this tea has been extensively used in traditional medicine across various cultures and is considered to possess potential anti-cancer properties.

Health Benefits and Anti-Cancer Potential

Graviola leaf tea is rich in antioxidants, which help neutralize free radicals in the body and protect cells from damage. This attribute suggests it may contribute to cancer prevention and offer complementary support. Its anti-inflammatory properties aid in alleviating chronic inflammation, enhancing immune system function, and strengthening the body's resistance to illness.

The anti-cancer potential of Graviola primarily stems from its bioactive compounds, such as acetogenins and annonacin. Experimental studies have indicated that these compounds may exhibit anti-tumor activity and inhibit the growth of cancer cells.

Beyond its possible anti-cancer effects, Graviola leaf tea is known for its calming properties, which can help reduce anxiety, alleviate stress, and improve sleep quality—factors particularly beneficial for individuals in recovery. In traditional medicine, it is also frequently used to combat infections and boost immunity, supporting overall health maintenance.

Consumption Guidelines and Precautions

A daily intake of 1 to 2 cups of Graviola leaf tea is generally considered appropriate. To minimize the risk of potential tolerance or side effects, it may be helpful to follow a routine of drinking the tea for three weeks, then taking a one-week break before continuing.

If symptoms such as nausea, headaches, or muscle cramps occur, consider reducing the consumption or discontinuing use, while closely monitoring the body's reactions.

This careful approach ensures that the potential benefits of Graviola leaf tea can be maximized while minimizing any risks.

Dandelion: Supporting Liver Health

Dandelion, a traditional medicinal herb and edible plant, is widely celebrated for its diverse health benefits. From its roots to its leaves and flowers, every part of the dandelion offers significant medicinal and nutritional value.

In the section on detox smoothies, we have already highlighted the benefits of combining dandelion with other fruits and vegetables. Additionally, dandelion is a staple in traditional Chinese medicine. Characterized as cooling in nature with a slightly bitter yet sweet taste, it is associated with the liver and stomach meridians. Dandelion is known for its diuretic, detoxifying, digestive, and anti-bloating properties. Regular consumption of dandelion tea or incorporating it into smoothies not only offers a refreshing taste but also helps to clear heat, detoxify the body, boost metabolism, and support the elimination of toxins, contributing to a healthier digestive system.

Below, we explore the specific health benefits of dandelion in greater detail:

1. Supporting Liver and Kidney Functions

Dandelion root is particularly valued for its natural detoxifying properties. It stimulates bile production in the liver, aiding in the breakdown and elimination of metabolic waste from the body. This process not only supports healthy liver function but also optimizes the overall performance of the digestive system. Moreover, the diuretic components in dandelion root promote urine production, facilitating the removal of toxins through the kidneys. This gentle detoxification process helps maintain internal balance, ensuring proper liver and kidney function while strengthening the entire detoxification system.

2. Anti-Inflammatory and Antioxidant Properties

Dandelion root possesses significant anti-inflammatory and antioxidant qualities, which contribute to bolstering the immune system. Its rich antioxidants help neutralize free radicals in the body, reducing cellular damage. This makes it an important component in cancer prevention and recovery support.

3. Cancer Prevention and Recovery Support

Research suggests that dandelion root extract may have the potential to inhibit the growth of certain cancer cells and promote their apoptosis (programmed cell death). Fresh dandelion root can be dried through slow simmering and prepared as a tea, a method believed to release its active compounds more effectively and enhance its anti-cancer properties.

By incorporating dandelion into your routine, whether as tea or in other forms, you can support liver detoxification, boost immune function, and potentially benefit from its cancer-protective effects.

Consumption Guidelines and Precautions

For individuals with sensitive stomachs, consuming dandelion tea on an empty stomach may not be suitable. It may be helpful to drink the tea about 30 minutes after meals to support stomach health, as drinking it on an empty stomach could potentially irritate the gastric lining and lead to discomfort.

When used appropriately, dandelion offers a natural and effective way to support liver health, enhance overall well-being, and contribute to long-term health maintenance.

Additional Support Strategies: A Multidimensional Approach

Among the various integrated strategies, the following three therapies have also played a significant role in our journey to combat cancer. These therapies, combined with others, are designed to enhance overall recovery outcomes.

Next, we will explore in depth how these therapies provide multifaceted support throughout this process.

Cautious Vaccination: A Strategy For Immune Balance

When considering alternative therapies as a means of supporting cancer recovery, it is often recommended to delay vaccination during the healing process. This is because certain vaccines may place additional strain on an immune system already weakened by cancer and its treatments. It is important to approach this decision under the guidance of a medical professional to ensure it does not negatively impact the recovery process.

Based on my personal experience, completely avoiding vaccination during this period proved crucial. Consequently, both Yulia and I refrained from receiving any vaccines.

The specific reasons are as follows:

1. Fragility of the Immune System

The immune systems of individuals affected by cancer are often highly compromised, with significantly reduced resilience. In such a state, the efficacy and safety of vaccines are difficult to evaluate and may result in unpredictable side effects. This is particularly true in severe stages of cancer, such as during metastasis, where vaccination might trigger severe complications and further compromise overall health.

2. Potential Effects of Vaccines

In some cases, vaccination could interfere with the recovery process facilitated by natural therapies, increasing the risk of adverse reactions or disrupting overall bodily regulation. Due to the immune system's potential dysfunction caused by the disease, vaccines may occasionally overactivate the immune system, leading to unpredictable health responses. Furthermore, the potential side effects of vaccines could complicate the recovery journey.

3. Careful Assessment of Vaccination

For cancer-affected individuals who have opted for natural therapies and paused conventional treatments, particularly those with highly vulnerable immune systems, it is crucial to carefully assess the necessity and potential risks of vaccination. Weighing the pros and cons comprehensively is essential to ensure that all interventions support overall health and recovery without imposing additional burdens or potential adverse effects on the immune system.

Mini Trampoline: Enhancing Lymphatic Flow

The up-and-down bouncing motion on a mini trampoline is regarded as an effective way to stimulate lymphatic drainage. It activates fascial tissues, helps eliminate waste and toxins from the body, strengthens the immune system, and provides substantial support during the recovery process.

Key Benefits for Cancer Recovery

1. The Importance of the Lymphatic System

The lymphatic system plays a critical role in removing toxins and waste from the body. Unlike the heart, the lymphatic system lacks a pump to drive lymph fluid flow. The rhythmic compression of lymphatic vessels achieved through bouncing on a mini trampoline promotes lymph flow and facilitates natural detoxification. This gentle form of exercise is particularly beneficial for a lymphatic system weakened by illness, helping it gradually regain normal function.

2. Improved Blood Circulation

In addition to enhancing lymphatic drainage, the gentle bouncing motion effectively improves overall blood circulation. The vertical movement supports the cardiovascular system, allowing oxygen and nutrients to be delivered more efficiently throughout the body while aiding rapid blood return to the heart. By promoting optimal lymphatic and blood flow, this activity reduces systemic inflammation, strengthens immune function, and equips the body to better combat infections and diseases.

3. Stress Relief

Mini trampoline exercises are both gentle and effective, helping to reduce overactivity of the sympathetic nervous system and encouraging deep relaxation throughout the body. During exercise, endorphins (the "feel-good hormones") are released, improving mood and alleviating stress caused by cancer or other health challenges. This contributes to an overall uplift in mental well-being.

Safety and Adaptability

When using a mini trampoline to promote lymphatic drainage, it is important to select an appropriate intensity level based on individual health and fitness levels to ensure both safety and effectiveness. A simple, low-impact routine of just 15 minutes a day can yield significant benefits. During exercise, focus on relaxed, controlled movements, avoiding excessive force to achieve daily detoxification without placing undue stress on the body.

Regularly engaging in this gentle activity not only helps prevent muscle loss but also maintains or enhances physical strength, particularly during recovery. By promoting lymphatic drainage, improving blood circulation, relieving stress, and boosting immune function, mini trampoline exercises offer robust support for comprehensive recovery.

Cannabis Oil: A Natural Hope In The Fight Against Cancer

THC (tetrahydrocannabinol), the primary active ingredient in cannabis oil, has garnered significant attention in recent years for its potential anti-cancer effects. Studies suggest that THC may limit tumor growth by inducing apoptosis (programmed cell death) in cancer cells and inhibiting tumor angiogenesis. Additionally, THC is recognized for its anti-inflammatory and appetite-stimulating properties, as well as its calming, anti-anxiety, and antidepressant effects. These benefits make it particularly suitable for cancer patients experiencing insomnia caused by pain, stress, or anxiety. When used appropriately, THC can reduce the time needed to fall asleep, improve sleep quality, and effectively alleviate physical and emotional discomfort.

Given the diverse potential benefits of THC, cannabis oil has been recognized in certain studies as a promising alternative therapy, particularly for alleviating cancer-related pain and inhibiting tumor growth. However, it is important to emphasize that these studies remain in the early stages, and individual responses to treatment may vary significantly. Furthermore, the legality of THC differs across countries and regions, making it essential to thoroughly understand the applicable local laws before use. In countries such as Canada, specific states in the United States, and Germany, THC has been approved for medical purposes, though its use is strictly regulated. Conversely, in other regions, THC may be entirely prohibited. In jurisdictions where its use is permitted, THC cannabis oil can be obtained through pharmacies, specialized retailers, or authorized suppliers. It is critical to ensure that products are sourced from reputable providers and used under the guidance of qualified medical professionals to prevent misuse.

Guidelines for Using THC

A dose of THC cannabis oil about the size of a grain of rice, taken nightly, is recommended for safe use to help improve sleep and promote recovery. If THC is not legally available in your country or region, you may refer to other natural therapies discussed in this book, which can also support health and recovery.

It is important to note that THC is a complementary therapy among various approaches to managing cancer and should not be regarded as the sole or primary treatment method.

Integrated Therapies: The Essence of Anti-Cancer Strength

The therapies described earlier have provided invaluable support and significant positive effects in our fight against cancer. They emphasize holistic mind-body adjustments, focusing on long-term recovery and health management. By enhancing the body's self-healing capacity and promoting internal and external balance, these approaches elevate overall therapeutic outcomes. These therapies not only support physical recovery but also serve as a source of hope and life transformation.

Summary of Key Elements in These Therapies

1. Lifestyle and Nutrition

Adjusting lifestyle habits and managing diet are crucial in this journey. Proper nutrition provides the energy required for bodily repair and resilience, while effective stress management lays the foundation for restoring balance and promoting recovery. Together, these measures significantly accelerate the body's natural healing processes.

2. Hydration and Health Support

Water, the essence of life, becomes an even more vital pillar during recovery. Adequate hydration is critical for maintaining kidney health and supporting immune system function. Water aids in flushing out toxins, boosting metabolism, and alleviating common side effects of recovery, such as fatigue and nausea, helping the body maintain balance more effectively.

3. Kidney Function and Detoxification

The kidneys, as primary detoxifying organs, play a key role in removing metabolic waste and toxins while maintaining fluid balance and indirectly supporting immune system function. Accumulated toxins can strain the kidneys, making their protection essential. Enhancing detoxification capabilities reduces toxic reactions and accelerates recovery. The coordinated functions of the liver and kidneys create a strong detoxification barrier, providing robust support for the body's healing process.

4. pH Balance and Internal Environment

Maintaining the body's acid-base balance is a fundamental principle of natural therapies. Alkaline diets and regulation can help balance pH levels, creating an environment less conducive to cancer cell growth. This balance not only inhibits the spread of cancer cells but also fosters recovery and improves overall health. Thus, acid-base equilibrium forms the foundation of health and is central to the effectiveness of natural therapies.

5. Exercise and Mental Health

Exercise accelerates metabolism, aiding toxin elimination and stabilizing the internal environment. Beyond physical strength, exercise promotes the release of endorphins, improving mood, alleviating anxiety and stress, and enhancing psychological resilience. Mental well-being is integral to the entire cancer-fighting journey. The next chapter delves into how psychological adjustment and emotional support can amplify anti-cancer efforts. Therefore, exercise serves as both a booster for physical recovery and a cornerstone of mental restoration.

6. Sleep and Immune Support

Quality sleep is essential for self-repair and immune system support. During sleep, the body regenerates cells, restores the immune system, and regulates hormones—processes critical for health and disease resistance. Furthermore, a regular sleep schedule and a healthy gut microbiome work together to strengthen the immune system. Consuming probiotic-rich fermented foods and increasing vitamin D levels through sunlight exposure are effective ways to enhance this function. Thus, sleep is the cornerstone of recovery and an essential safeguard for mind and body rejuvenation.

7. Patience, Belief, and Sustainability

The benefits of natural therapies often require time to accumulate. Patience, emotional stability, and persistence are vital throughout the recovery process. With continuous self-healing support, the body enters a gradual process of returning to health. Personalized recovery plans and ongoing adjustments can effectively restore balance, promoting long-term vitality and health. The enduring effects of these therapies stem from steadfast commitment, forming the foundation for sustainable recovery.

8. Synergistic Effects

The integrated application of natural therapies aims to comprehensively enhance the body's self-regulation and healing capacities. Through the interplay of multiple therapies, a well-structured recovery strategy achieves synergistic effects, helping the body establish a healthy internal environment and significantly boosting cellular self-repair functions. This comprehensive approach builds a solid foundation for long-term health, supporting sustained well-being. Additionally, psychological balance and emotional stability are indispensable aspects of the recovery process. Thus, the combined application of these therapies plays a pivotal role in the journey to recovery.

Conclusion

The therapies introduced in this chapter not only yield noticeable recovery results in the short term but also provide a sustainable approach to long-term health management. Each therapy has its unique benefits, and their combined application can significantly enhance overall effectiveness, offering comprehensive support throughout the recovery process. These methods integrate the scientific foundation of modern medicine with the essence of wisdom found in traditional herbal and natural therapies. Tailored adjustments and regular monitoring based on individual needs ensure optimal outcomes, paving a steady path to recovery.

The success of these integrative therapies not only grants us a renewed chance at life but also serves as a valuable guide for maintaining long-term health. Even after recovery, these therapies remain an essential part of sustaining well-being. Personally, I have intermittently incorporated these methods into my daily life, and over nearly a decade since then, I have not required medical attention due to illness. These strategies are not only beneficial in the fight against cancer but also serve as a reference for anyone striving for health and longevity. Consistent practice of these approaches lays a solid foundation for lasting well-being.

These therapies are like a beacon of light in the darkness, guiding us forward, opening a new chapter in the journey back to health, and setting the wheel of life in motion once more. They enable us to continue enjoying and experiencing the vibrant world around us. We are also eager to share these invaluable experiences with others in need, hoping that they, too, can draw inspiration, regain confidence, and find strength on their path to health.

CHUNMEI YAO

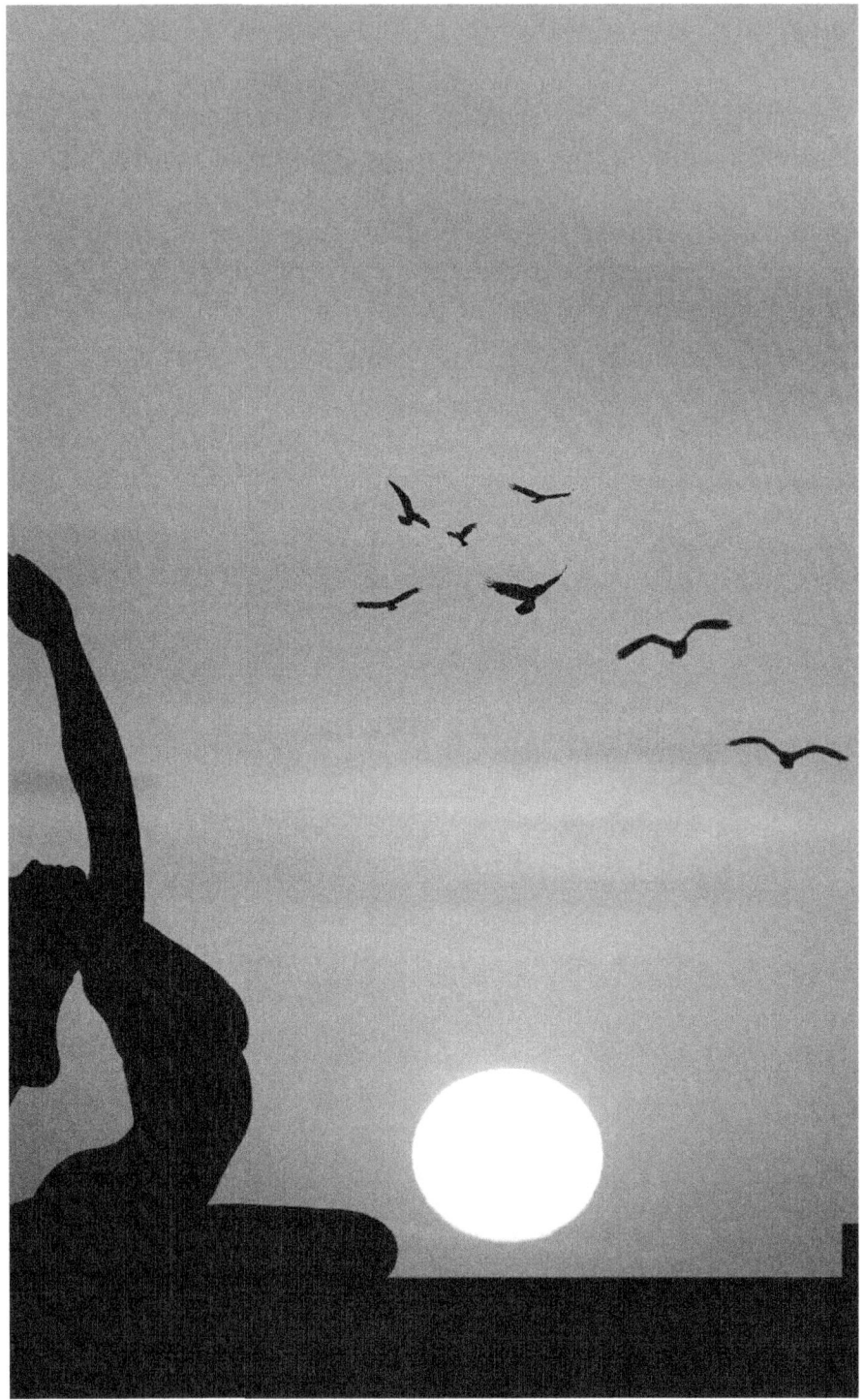

CHAPTER 6: THE POWER OF THE MIND – EMOTIONAL SUPPORT AND A VICTORIOUS MENTALITY

In the previous chapter, we detailed the various strategies Julia and I employed during our battle against cancer—approaches that played a pivotal role in our recovery. However, to truly overcome cancer, the strength of the mind and emotions must not be overlooked. These inner forces not only directly influence the recovery process but also profoundly affect the pace of healing and overall quality of life. By strengthening mental health, effectively managing stress, and fostering positive emotions and attitudes, individuals can better navigate the challenges of illness and promote holistic recovery.

Some individuals live a tranquil life before receiving a cancer diagnosis, but upon learning of their condition, they quickly spiral into emotional collapse, leading to a rapid decline in physical health and, ultimately, loss of life. Such tragedies highlight the inseparable connection between mental and physical well-being. When the psyche is shattered, the body can scarcely endure, and even the most effective treatments may lose their potency. The mind serves as a bridge between the body and spirit—a convergence point for mental and physical resilience.

Conversely, there are those who, after diagnosis, let go of previous obsessions, choose to reconnect with nature, breathe fresh air, travel to new places, or experience untried adventures—and astonishingly recover. Such cases are not uncommon. When people consciously release mental burdens, open their hearts, embrace their true emotions, and establish a more natural and harmonious relationship with themselves and the world around them, stress gradually dissipates. This psychological "unbinding" allows individuals to return to a natural state, where both body and mind find relaxation and balance.

In this state, the body releases more "happiness hormones" like endorphins and serotonin, which not only elevate mood and alleviate pain but also enhance immune function. Simultaneously, inner calm reduces anxiety and stress responses, enabling the body to focus more effectively on self-repair. In essence, this relaxed and natural state is not merely a psychological adjustment but a path to holistic harmony that positively impacts the stress associated with cancer. It further underscores the importance of mental and emotional strength in the fight against cancer. A joyful mind is the best "medicine" for recovery, and a positive attitude often determines whether one chooses hope or succumbs to despair when facing adversity.

Thus, inner strength not only influences how one confronts the challenges of illness but also shapes their ability to approach recovery and its side effects with optimism. This strength helps individuals maintain confidence and perseverance in adversity, enabling them to navigate uncertainties and difficulties with composure. Only by consciously cultivating inner strength can one better endure physical discomfort, find psychological support, and rise to every challenge.

This truth resonates deeply with me. After my physical recovery, many people reached out to ask how I managed to overcome cancer successfully. I always shared my experiences openly. While some achieved miraculous recoveries through these strategies, others did not succeed. Through careful observation, I realized that these differences were often closely tied to the individuals' mental preparedness and emotional states. The profound connection between mental health and the cancer journey is precisely why this chapter focuses on this critical topic.

As mentioned in Chapter 5, a positive belief system can create effects similar to the placebo effect, representing a practical application of the law of attraction and a key to health. Medical research indicates that in some cases, this effect has a success rate of up to 50%, particularly concerning psychological and perceptual symptoms. This suggests that even without specific medications, the body can achieve partial self-healing through its intrinsic "pharmacological response." This phenomenon illustrates that beliefs and attitudes influence not only emotions and psychological states but also the physical recovery process directly.

At the core of the placebo effect lies subconscious self-suggestion. Conscious thought can influence the subconscious, which in turn governs most of the body's functions. Thus, during this critical period, positive psychological reinforcement is vital for the recovery journey. Indeed, the power of the mind and emotions can sometimes surpass that of medicine. With this understanding, we hope all those affected by cancer will recognize the significance of mental and emotional strength and view it as an essential pillar in their journey to healing.

Next, we will delve deeper into the pivotal role of emotional strength in this journey:

Stress Management: Key Strategies and Methods

When faced with a significant challenge like cancer, the mind often becomes overwhelmed with fear, anxiety, and a sense of pressure. These negative emotions can place the body in a prolonged "stress state," increasing psychological burdens while potentially compromising the immune system's normal functions. This can delay healing and hinder the body's ability to repair itself. Without effective stress management, these burdens may escalate, leading to emotional instability such as irritability, anger, and confusion, while exacerbating inflammatory responses.

On the other hand, effective stress management strategies can help individuals better navigate the psychological and physical challenges of their cancer journey, thereby increasing the likelihood of recovery. Stress management is not only essential for emotional stability but also plays a critical role in supporting the body's natural healing processes. By employing healthy emotional management techniques, individuals can acknowledge and accept emotional fluctuations, reduce the negative impact of emotions on their mind and body, and strengthen their ability to cope with stress.

Here are some key strategies and methods:

Nutrition And Self-Care

A healthy diet plays a crucial role in managing, coping with, and alleviating stress. Balanced nutrition helps regulate hormone levels, particularly stress-related hormones like cortisol. Foods rich in complex carbohydrates, such as whole grains, provide steady energy and help prevent blood sugar fluctuations, thereby reducing mood swings caused by stress. Additionally, foods high in omega-3 fatty acids, such as fish and nuts, help reduce inflammation and support neurotransmitter balance, which can mitigate stress responses. Nutrients like B vitamins and magnesium further contribute to the proper functioning of the nervous system, enhancing the body's resilience to stress. Scientific research also demonstrates that nutritional status directly affects the body's ability to manage stress, while prolonged stress can impair nutrient absorption and utilization. During cancer recovery, the body's nutritional demands increase significantly. A nutrient-rich diet not only boosts immune function but also helps the body better combat cancer and reduce the risk of recurrence.

Sleep

Quality sleep is an indispensable component of stress management. Stress often disrupts sleep quality, and poor sleep exacerbates psychological stress, creating a vicious cycle. By ensuring restorative sleep, individuals can better regulate stress and support the body's natural healing processes.

Time Management And Life Planning

Maintaining a structured daily routine is particularly important. Effective time management is one of the key factors in alleviating stress. A well-organized schedule that balances work and rest not only aids physical recovery but also reduces uncertainties in life, fostering a sense of control. For example, during my illness, I had to manage daily cancer treatments and related tasks while simultaneously running a business and overseeing various aspects of a house-building project. This tightly packed schedule left little room for stress or sadness, allowing me to remain focused and emotionally stable most of the time. I firmly believe that proactive life planning was a crucial factor in my successful recovery.

Goal Setting And Planning

Clear values and goals provide inner motivation and a positive mindset, enabling individuals to focus on action and achievement rather than dwelling on negative emotions. Goals also instill a sense of control, especially during challenging times, offering guidance and support.

Breaking down clear and actionable goals into small, manageable steps creates a continuous sense of accomplishment. This structured approach not only fosters a sense of autonomy but also effectively alleviates anxiety and stress. For instance, during the house construction phase of my illness, I never worried about what would happen if my health declined. Instead, I lived and worked according to a predetermined plan, which gave me a sense of fulfillment rather than being consumed by my illness. Focusing on concrete goals significantly reduced negative emotions and further strengthened my confidence and chances of overcoming cancer.

Physical Activity

Although cancer treatments may cause fatigue, gentle exercises like tai chi, qigong, walking, and yoga can effectively restore energy. These low-intensity activities help maintain physical vitality, promote blood circulation, enhance immune function, and release endorphins that alleviate stress and improve mood.

Emotional Processing

Creative outlets for emotional expression, such as art, writing, painting, or music, help relax the mind and release inner feelings. Journaling is an effective way to clarify thoughts and relieve stress, offering a means to maintain emotional balance. These activities not only reduce the impact of negative emotions but also help individuals focus and express their feelings constructively.

Mindfulness Practices

Mindfulness, meditation, and deep breathing exercises are powerful tools for reducing stress and enhancing psychological resilience, as discussed in Chapter 5. These techniques enable individuals to focus on the present moment, freeing them from worries about the unknown or uncertainties of the future. Mindfulness and deep breathing help regulate emotions, reduce attachment to negative thoughts, and enhance self-awareness. Combining mindfulness with deep breathing not only alleviates stress and improves sleep but also strengthens the body's self-healing abilities.

Individual Differences

Every person responds differently to stress management strategies. Therefore, it is essential to tailor stress management plans to individual circumstances and select the most suitable methods. Personalized strategies are more effective in meeting individual needs, improving the overall effectiveness of stress management. Consistently practicing appropriate stress management techniques is vital for maintaining long-term physical and mental well-being.

By employing these multi-dimensional stress management strategies, individuals can face the challenges of cancer recovery with greater composure, maintain a positive mindset, and enhance their physical and emotional resilience. Integrating stress management into the overall fight against disease not only significantly improves quality of life but also lays a solid foundation for lasting health.

Mental Health: An Essential Pillar

A healthy mental state not only boosts immunity but also significantly enhances the likelihood of successful recovery. Research shows that psychological well-being and personality traits can influence health to a certain extent. When facing cancer, individuals often endure immense physical and emotional stress, including fear of the recovery process, anxiety about the future, and impacts on self-esteem. In such circumstances, psychological support becomes especially crucial. By strengthening mental resilience, adaptability, and stress-coping mechanisms, individuals can better navigate these challenges. Positive psychological interventions not only stabilize emotions but also promote the body's self-repair mechanisms, thereby improving overall recovery outcomes and health levels.

The critical role of mental health can be summarized in the following aspects :

The Power Of Belief And Hope

Mental and emotional strength plays a decisive role in maintaining hope and self-motivation. A positive mindset helps set realistic and achievable goals while fostering optimism about the future, which is particularly critical during the recovery process. Even in the most challenging moments, a strong sense of belief can help individuals find meaning in life, inspiring proactive actions to promote healing. This belief not only alleviates psychological stress but also strengthens immune function, enhancing the body's ability to combat illness.

Emotional Regulation, Resilience, And Recovery

Emotional regulation is essential in addressing fear, sadness, and anger that often accompany a cancer diagnosis. Healthy emotional processing allows individuals to acknowledge and accept these feelings without being overwhelmed, while simultaneously building psychological resilience and recovery capacity. Robust emotional resilience enables individuals to remain calm and focused under physical and emotional stress, thus facilitating the recovery process. Enhanced adaptability further helps individuals navigate changes during recovery, fostering confidence and a sense of control over uncertainties.

Nutrition

Proper nutrition is crucial in this journey, not only for strengthening physical endurance and recovery capacity but also for supporting normal brain function, which influences mood and cognitive performance. As the body grows stronger, maintaining a positive, balanced, and relaxed state becomes easier, enabling individuals to cope with stress effectively and preserve mental well-being. Research indicates that diets rich in fruits, vegetables, whole grains, and lean proteins can reduce the risk of depression and anxiety. These diets, abundant in antioxidants, help reduce inflammation and protect brain health. Amino acids in proteins, such as tryptophan, contribute to the production of serotonin, the "happiness hormone," stabilizing mood. Furthermore, the intake of vitamin D, B vitamins, and omega-3 fatty acids is closely linked to improved mood and cognitive function. Therefore, a healthy diet not only benefits physical health but also effectively supports mental well-being, fostering a positive and balanced mindset. These two aspects complement and reinforce each other.

Sleep

Quality sleep is the foundation of the body's repair capabilities. During deep sleep, growth hormones are released, promoting cellular regeneration and tissue repair. A healthy psychological state improves sleep quality, supporting the body's self-healing processes. Establishing a healthy sleep pattern not only enhances cognitive function and emotional stability but also improves overall quality of life. Together, good mental health and high-quality sleep underpin the body's ability to heal itself, providing critical support for overcoming illness.

Recovery Outcomes

Studies have shown that good mental health significantly enhances recovery outcomes. A positive psychological state and strong willpower enable individuals to exhibit greater adherence to treatment plans, achieving better therapeutic results.

Integrating mental health into a comprehensive recovery plan fosters balance and harmony between mind and body. This holistic approach not only improves psychological and physical recovery but also equips individuals to handle illness more effectively through psychological therapy, emotional support, and the cultivation of spiritual strength. Additionally, spiritual experiences play a vital role in mental health, offering comfort, hope, and fulfillment of spiritual needs. These experiences provide emotional support and motivation, creating a holistic recovery perspective that underscores the importance of mental health and reveals the positive impact of spiritual well-being on recovery.

Such a comprehensive strategy helps individuals maintain a positive mindset and strong inner strength when facing the challenges of illness. Mental health is not only an essential pillar in the fight against cancer but also the cornerstone of holistic recovery. By integrating these mental health strategies, individuals can maintain steadfast beliefs and receive emotional support, achieving the goal of comprehensive recovery.

In summary, the role of mental health in the cancer recovery process cannot be underestimated. It provides both emotional and spiritual support while aiding individuals in developing greater resilience and adaptability when facing challenges through effective psychological regulation. Additionally, a positive psychological state strengthens immune function and supports the body's self-repair mechanisms, laying the foundation for better recovery outcomes. Comprehensive mental health management helps individuals achieve balance and strength during recovery, enhancing quality of life and paving the way toward sustained health.

Stress and Mental Health: Interconnection and Balance

In the previous sections, we explored the critical roles of stress management and mental health during this challenging period. As key components of emotional support, these two aspects are closely interconnected. They not only have a profound impact on the recovery process but also hold extraordinary significance for long-term overall health.

The Key Connections Between Stress Management and Mental Health

Stress And Mental Health Challenges

Failing to effectively manage and release stress over the long term can lead to mental health issues, adversely affecting overall quality of life. For individuals already experiencing mental health challenges, stress can exacerbate symptoms, making the situation more complex and difficult to control, thereby hindering the recovery process. As noted at the conclusion of Chapter 4, alleviating stress can accelerate psychological recovery, enabling individuals to emerge from difficulties more quickly and maintain mental balance.

Mental Health Enhancing Stress Management

A positive mental health state enhances an individual's ability to cope with stress. When mental well-being is maintained, individuals are more likely to adopt active and effective strategies for addressing challenges. Improved mental health also reduces sensitivity to stressors and diminishes the perceived intensity of stress. For those struggling to self-regulate stress or manage negative emotions, seeking professional psychological support can be an effective approach.

In summary, Stress management and mental health are deeply interconnected, mutually reinforcing one another to cultivate a positive state of mind and body. Enhanced psychological balance and resilience empower individuals to respond to stress with greater composure and effectiveness, leading to better decision-making and improved overall outcomes. Together, these factors create a foundation for navigating challenges with strength and stability.

Support from Loved Ones: The Warmth and Strength of Companionship

As previously discussed, mental health and stress management are vital pillars during this journey, and the support of family and friends plays a crucial role alongside them. Their presence offers not only emotional comfort but also practical assistance, serving as a powerful foundation for both psychological and physical recovery. For instance, during my illness, their care provided me with emotional solace and meticulous help in daily life, further strengthening my resolve to fight cancer. Their unwavering support became the most reliable pillar of my journey, profoundly influencing my emotions and quality of life while significantly bolstering my mental resilience. It was an indispensable source of strength in overcoming challenges.

The following are specific ways in which they supported me throughout this process:

Spiritual And Emotional Support

My family and friends provided me with immense spiritual and emotional support. During my most painful moments, they sat with me, reminiscing over cherished memories captured in photos and videos, evoking positive feelings that temporarily eased my suffering and comforted my heart. They also encouraged me to participate in family activities, allowing me to feel warmth and strength while ensuring that my life was not entirely disrupted by illness. This helped me maintain a positive and optimistic outlook, solidifying my resolve to face cancer with courage.

We often went for walks together, especially in nature, which helped me step out of the shadow of illness. Whenever I needed them, they were always by my side without hesitation, making me feel deeply secure and never alone or helpless. They patiently listened to my concerns, closely monitored my recovery progress, and provided unwavering understanding and compassion. This alleviated my inner stress and unease, significantly reducing my anxiety and fostering emotional resilience.

Practical Support

In daily life, my family and friends took on many responsibilities, such as shopping, cooking, cleaning, and coordinating various schedules, ensuring that I attended follow-up appointments on time. These practical contributions greatly alleviated the burden of daily life, allowing me to focus more energy on my recovery. They drove me to hospital visits, helped interpret the doctors' advice, and shared insights with me, making me feel endlessly supported.

Respect And Dignity

Throughout their care, my family and friends always respected my preferences and decisions, ensuring that I never felt stripped of my autonomy. This respect allowed me to maintain a sense of control and confidence during the most challenging times, which was invaluable to me.

Gratitude From The Heart

I am filled with gratitude for my family and friends. Their understanding and companionship became my most vital source of strength during this difficult period, enabling me to persevere. In the future, when they need my support, I will not hesitate to be there for them, repaying the endless love and warmth they have shown me.

In summary, the emotional and practical support provided by my family, friends, and support network was indispensable. It greatly enhanced my mental resilience and self-healing capabilities. This robust network of support helped me maintain an optimistic mindset and laid a strong foundation for my recovery, guiding me toward a healthier and happier future.

Conclusion

In this chapter, we delved into the critical roles of stress management, mental health, and social support in the journey of battling cancer, highlighting how these factors strengthen psychological resilience. Confronting the challenges of cancer, I learned to reduce emotional fluctuations through stress management and effective time planning, maintaining inner peace and focus. A stable routine not only helped me steer clear of unnecessary anxiety but also served as a "remedy" during this difficult period. Regardless of the uncertainties the future may hold, spiritual strength has remained my steadfast pillar, empowering me to move forward with courage.

In summary, inner strength, emotional support, and a robust social support system enabled me to face numerous challenges with composure and ultimately achieve recovery. I hope my experiences provide valuable insights and encouragement to those navigating similar struggles.

CHUNMEI YAO

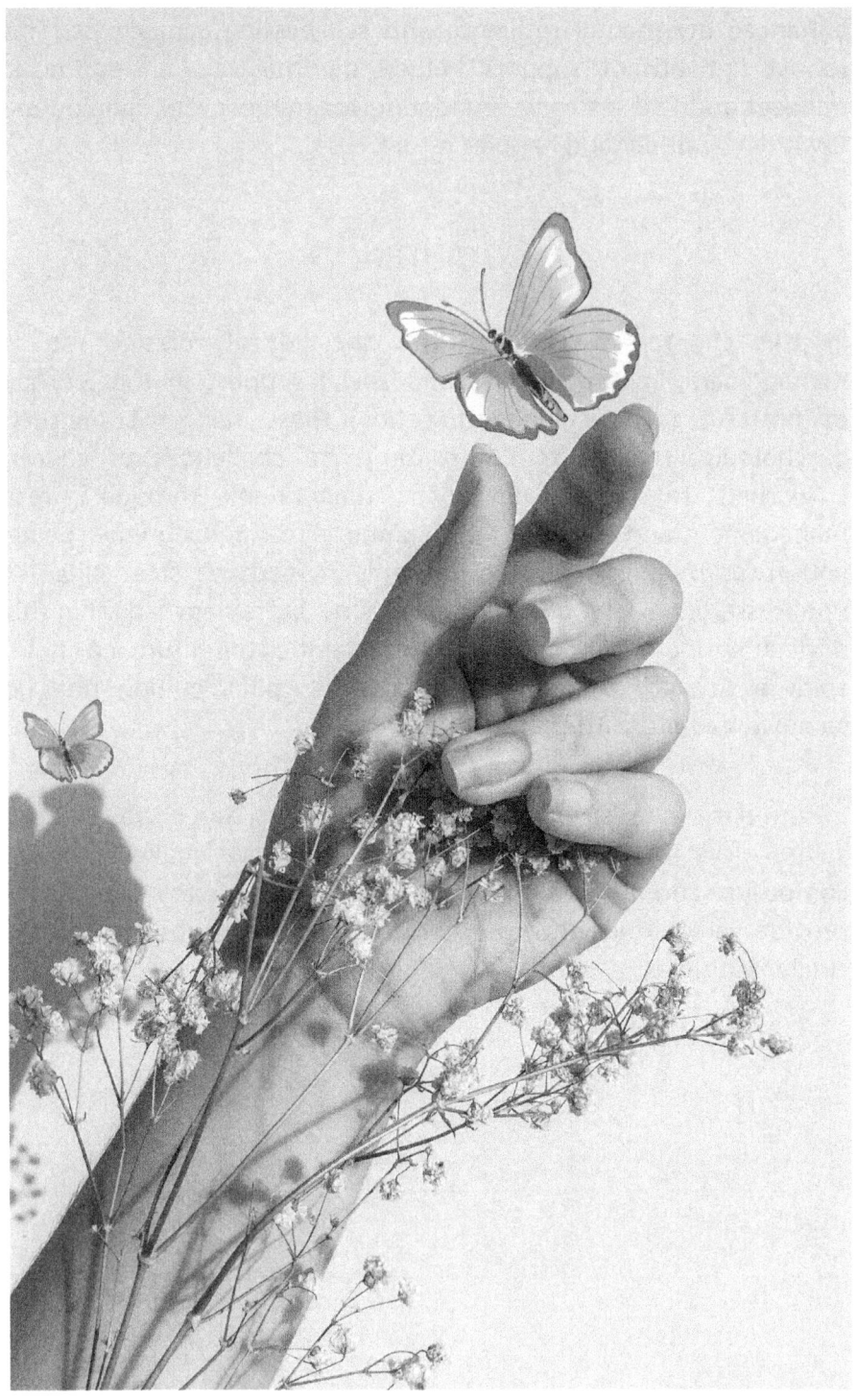

CHAPTER 7: THE PATH TO RECOVERY – REAL STORIES AND REFLECTIONS

In the previous two chapters, we explored various healing methods and strategies that played a decisive role in physical recovery. This chapter shifts focus to the emotional journey within this process. The path to recovery is not merely about physical healing but also the rebirth of the soul. Each stage brought profound transformations for both body and mind, allowing me to rediscover the priceless nature of life. These challenging moments, though painful, fostered an inner strength I had never experienced before, enabling me to face life's uncertainties with unwavering determination.

In the darkest depths of my life, the only thing that guided me was my vision for the future. A faint yet resolute light pierced through the heavy fog, illuminating my path forward. It was more than just a glimmer of hope—it was a force, a reminder that life still held promise. This belief was what kept me from giving up during the most difficult days. I firmly believed that no matter how daunting the road ahead might be, perseverance would eventually lead me to my own miracle and a new dawn.

For my family and me, hope marked the starting point of this recovery journey. It became an intangible yet powerful force embedded in every decision and every seemingly insignificant choice we made. As I gradually learned to accept the imperfections of reality, my fears and anxieties were replaced by steadfast confidence and fearless resolve. This shift allowed me to transition from passively enduring the recovery process to actively embracing every rise and fall, every change in life. I came to realize that this journey was not just about regaining health but also about my inner transformation.

After months of emotional upheaval and uncertainty, I finally witnessed the first positive sign. In that moment, the flame of hope within me reignited. I understood that this was not just physical recovery but a spiritual awakening—a newfound inner strength compelling me to keep moving forward. This pivotal moment became a significant turning point in my recovery, symbolizing the first rays of dawn breaking through the darkness. It marked not only the gradual restoration of physical health but also a leap in psychological growth and self-confidence. It taught me that every trial in life is a valuable lesson, and the strength gained from overcoming them becomes a lifelong companion.

Each person's path to recovery is unique, yet nearly every story of healing shares a common thread: a critical moment when a glimmer of hope quietly emerges, reigniting one's confidence. When this new direction appears, it becomes a guiding beacon in the recovery journey, signifying the transition from despair to hope, from illness to health. This is more than just physical restoration—it is a transformation from within. The strength derived from this transformation not only empowers us to confront illness but also instills in us the courage to embrace life fully. It allows us to greet each new day with hope and resilience, ready to face whatever challenges lie ahead.

Moments of Relief: Embracing Every Victory

The journey toward recovery felt like a long and grueling battle, with each day bringing new challenges. Every morning, I woke up to confront fatigue, pain, and a persistent fear deep within me. This struggle felt like an invisible shackle, weighing heavily on my heart, leaving me almost breathless. My strength was often depleted, and even the simplest daily tasks became dauntingly difficult.

Despite this, I insisted on going for walks every day, even though each step seemed to drain my remaining energy. On one occasion, my legs felt unbearably heavy, as if every step through the muddy ground was holding me back. Halfway through, I found myself completely exhausted, leaning against a large tree, torn between continuing forward or stopping and giving up. Every step felt like a burden pressing me into the ground, with fatigue casting a dark shadow over me. At that moment, from somewhere deep inside, a warm surge of energy slowly rose within me. It was like a faint but unyielding flame, gradually illuminating my dimming spirit. This newfound strength not only dispelled my physical exhaustion but also awakened a profound desire for life within me. Taking a deep breath, I steadied myself, feeling the warmth supporting me, and resumed my steps with renewed determination. In that moment, I wasn't just walking forward; I was engaging in an inner dialogue of resilience and perseverance. Eventually, I completed a route I once thought impossible due to my lack of strength.

I realized then that this was not merely a physical reaction or breakthrough but a manifestation of the inner strength that had been supporting me all along. This short yet meaningful journey gave me a new understanding of my untapped potential, making recovery no longer seem like an unreachable dream but a tangible goal that could be achieved step by step. It marked a significant inner victory, infusing me with unshakable faith to keep moving forward. While the process of physical recovery was slow, every small milestone became a triumph for me. These victories symbolized hope for healing and underscored my unwavering belief: I possessed the strength to conquer this illness.

On this path to recovery, I learned to focus on every small change. Each follow-up appointment brought both anticipation and apprehension as I awaited the doctor's results. On one occasion, when the doctor reviewed my test report, carefully examining each indicator, I could feel my heart pounding in my chest. When he finally told me that the tumor size had started to shrink, a surge of emotion overwhelmed me. Tears of joy and relief streamed down my face. That moment was not only a medical breakthrough but also a psychological triumph—a milestone on this arduous journey that reignited my hope for the future.

These moments of relief gave me not only a glimpse of recovery but also the motivation to persist. They reminded me that my efforts would eventually bear fruit. Every small improvement became invaluable, energizing me with new courage and reinforcing my determination to continue fighting.

Each moment of relief felt like a glimmer of light, igniting hope in the darkness and illuminating my path forward. The shrinking of the tumor, the easing of pain, the gradual weight gain, and the restoration of strength were all forces guiding me out of the shadows toward the light. Every easier breath, every restful night, and every morning I woke up feeling slightly more energized became crucial milestones in my battle against cancer, representing positive shifts. Even when these improvements were so subtle they were almost imperceptible, they flowed together like gentle streams, forming a steadfast force that carried me steadily forward, closer to the finish line of recovery.

Emotional Growth: Rebuilding Inner Strength

While physical recovery brought me immense confidence, I soon realized that this journey was far more than a physiological battle. It was not only a test of willpower but also a profound challenge to my emotional and spiritual resilience. Throughout the illness, I believed myself to be strong, yet I could not avoid the inevitable fluctuations in my emotions. At times, an indescribable loneliness would quietly creep in, making it feel as though no one could truly understand the weight of my pain. On certain nights, waves of anxiety, fear, and helplessness engulfed me, filling every corner of my heart. When I closed my eyes, my mind was often consumed by the uncertainties of an unclear future.

In Chapter 3, The Pillar of Strength, I mentioned how every night before bed, my son would give me a warm hug—something I eagerly anticipated each day. His embrace felt like a gentle current of warmth, dispelling the cold and loneliness that lingered in the darkness. One evening, however, I waited for his hug, but he didn't come. A subtle sense of loss arose, as though I had been deprived of a vital source of support. Quietly, I went to his room and found him sound asleep, a peaceful smile resting on his face—a smile that reflected pure contentment. As I stood by his bedside, gazing at him, an unexpected warmth and tranquility began to fill my heart.

In that moment, I realized something profound: perhaps he had already sensed that my body was gradually recovering and that I no longer needed his nightly hugs as a source of encouragement. His silent reassurance felt like an unspoken promise, as if he were subtly affirming that my recovery journey had quietly begun. Feeling the resonance of his tender heart, a wave of strength surged within me—not just from the physical progress I was making, but from the unspoken connection we shared, a mutual understanding that silently assured us both that I was on the path to health.

As my body steadily recovered, I experienced a critical moment of emotional and spiritual growth. There were countless times during my battle with cancer when I felt vulnerable and helpless, even doubting my ability to persevere. But my son's warm smile made me reevaluate my inner strength, reminding me that I was never fighting this battle alone—my family had been cheering me on every step of the way. This emotional epiphany restored my inner faith and strength, enabling me to confront the uncertainties of the future with renewed determination.

Through this emotional and spiritual journey, I came to understand that vulnerability is not a weakness, and accepting help from others does not equate to failure. During the darkest days, it was the selfless support and care of my family and friends that guided me through the most challenging times, becoming the warmest light in my heart. When I allowed myself to open up to them and candidly admit my vulnerabilities, I felt an overwhelming sense of liberation. This rebuilding of emotional strength taught me that human resilience comes not only from individual fortitude but also from the support and connection shared with others.

This spiritual growth not only carried me through the long journey of battling cancer but also made me more confident and composed in daily life. I no longer fear the trials of life, because I know that no matter how insurmountable the obstacles may seem, I possess the inner strength to overcome them. This transformation was not merely an emotional evolution but also a profound awakening of self-awareness. It has made me more resilient and has taught me to cherish the often-overlooked, delicate beauty of everyday life.

Cancer taught me that true strength stems from inner peace and resilience. I have learned to find hope amid fear and direction in moments of uncertainty. This growth is not just an emotional transformation but also a spiritual elevation. This experience has given me a renewed perspective on myself and the world around me. Now, I no longer fear the unknown future because I am confident that I have the courage and strength to overcome any challenge that lies ahead.

Personal Achievements and Milestones: Overcoming Challenges

On this journey of renewal, every small step forward felt like a stairway to a new life. Recovery was not just about physical healing but also a profound transformation of the soul. Every milestone, no matter how small, became an essential step toward health, igniting the light of hope along the way.

The initial achievements, though seemingly insignificant, brought unparalleled satisfaction. For instance, standing for longer periods with minimal pain, walking a full circle around the garden, or enjoying a complete meal for the first time—simple moments of daily life that had once been routine now became cherished goals to strive toward. Every small breakthrough felt like a step closer to recovery, filling me with indescribable joy and pride.

I vividly remember the first time I managed to prepare a simple breakfast on my own. The sense of accomplishment was so overwhelming that I was nearly moved to tears. Though the process was slow and every movement required utmost care, placing that breakfast on the table brought an unparalleled sense of triumph. It wasn't just a meal; it was a symbol of reclaiming control over my daily life, an affirmation that I was gradually regaining autonomy and dignity. Recovery wasn't just about defeating illness—it was about reclaiming mastery over my own existence.

As my physical health continued to improve, I began to re-engage in activities I loved, with gardening once again becoming a part of my life. Each time I saw the plants in my garden thriving under the sunlight, I felt a profound connection with nature. Their growth mirrored my own journey of recovery—every green leaf, every budding sprout, represented my rebirth. The plants I nurtured with care and persistence became a testament to my approach to healing both body and soul. Together, we grew, evolving through patience, dedication, and relentless effort. They witnessed each breakthrough and transformation, providing me with boundless strength and confidence.

What comforted me the most, however, was the gradual restoration of my social life. Illness had, at one point, forced me to distance myself from certain relationships. But now, I found my way back into the lives of those I cared about. Every reunion with friends, every conversation with family, became a pivotal moment in rediscovering the warmth of life. These heartfelt interactions reminded me that life is not just a solitary journey of resilience but also a tapestry of human connections. Sharing laughter, exchanging stories, and treasuring these precious moments brought me renewed faith in the power of relationships and the sense of safety they provide.

These personal achievements and milestones in recovery were more than just signs of physical improvement—they were reflections of my inner strength. Each small victory bore witness to my unwavering determination, a testament to the hope I had never relinquished. I understood that true success wasn't just about overcoming illness but about rediscovering every ounce of warmth in life and embracing its smallest details.

Now, more than ever, I appreciate the beauty of existence and the richness of daily life. The ordinary joys that emerged from this challenging journey have become my most valuable treasures. This profound sense of happiness, earned through perseverance, is the ultimate reward for everything I endured.

Reflection on the Journey of Healing: A Transformation from Darkness to Light

The journey of recovery was like a small tree growing resiliently through storms—each new leaf a tribute to life itself. The hardships I endured not only strengthened my resolve but also taught me how to embrace uncertainty with inner peace and move forward with steady steps, ready to face each new tomorrow. Looking back on this journey, I deeply feel that I have undergone a profound transformation from darkness to light. Each challenge, each turning point, is a mark of growth for both my mind and body. From the initial despair to gradually regaining hope and strength, every step along the way has shaped the strong and mature person I am today.

I vividly remember the moment I was diagnosed with late-stage cancer—it felt as though time had frozen. The doctor's words cut through me like a sharp blade, each one piercing deep into my heart. In an instant, the trajectory of my life was rewritten, and the future became distant and unfamiliar. Yet, despite being engulfed by fear and despair, I quickly realized that allowing negative emotions to consume me would not change my reality. As long as life persisted, I had to fight courageously and refuse to give up. I told myself that instead of being paralyzed by fear, I would give my all to seize every glimmer of hope. And so, with unwavering determination and relentless effort, I gradually overcame cancer.

Reflecting on this journey, I have come to understand that true healing is not solely dependent on medical advancements but also relies on the emotional support of loved ones and the strength of inner conviction. It was these supports that helped me reexamine the true value of life and equipped me with greater resilience and calmness in the face of adversity. Healing is not merely about physical recovery; it is also about the rebirth of the soul.

This journey, full of trials, has given me a deeper appreciation of life and health. It taught me patience and perseverance, and in my darkest moments, I glimpsed faint rays of light. Now, I understand that although the future may still be fraught with challenges, as long as hope resides in my heart, I have an inexhaustible source of strength to move forward with courage. I no longer fear the unknown, instead drawing strength from the wellsprings of faith and love.

In every low point, I learned how to summon courage, how to draw warmth from moments of love, and how to march forward with unwavering determination. This journey of healing not only helped me overcome illness but also revealed the resilience and brilliance of life itself. It has shaped a stronger, more fulfilled version of myself, ready to embrace whatever lies ahead.

Conclusion

In this chapter, we reflected on the arduous journey from the depths of illness to reclaiming health. The narrative captures the dual growth of body and mind throughout the recovery process—each incremental step of physical progress and every confrontation with inner fears and loneliness are testaments to unwavering willpower and profound emotional transformation. This journey was not merely a fight against disease but also a reformation of the soul.

We highlighted the pivotal role of family, friends, and spiritual pillars during this process. Their support and encouragement ensured that the path to healing extended beyond medical interventions, encompassing the warmth of emotional connections and the strength of faith. By continuously pushing personal boundaries, overcoming countless challenges, and gradually regaining physical health, this journey also fostered a profound awakening of the spirit. These experiences revealed that true strength lies not only in physical recovery but also in the accumulation of inner peace and resilience.

Ultimately, this journey instilled a more positive and composed mindset toward embracing every moment of life. At its core, recovery is not only about conquering illness but also about drawing strength from the details of everyday life and learning to re-embrace the essence of existence. This rebirth conveys themes of perseverance and the appreciation of life, reminding us that no matter how dark the moment, as long as there is light within our hearts, we can move toward new hope and brightness.

This experience deepened my understanding of the meaning of life, making me stronger and more at peace. It also prompted a thorough reassessment of all aspects of my life moving forward. In the chapters to come, we will delve further into these reflections and explore them in greater depth.

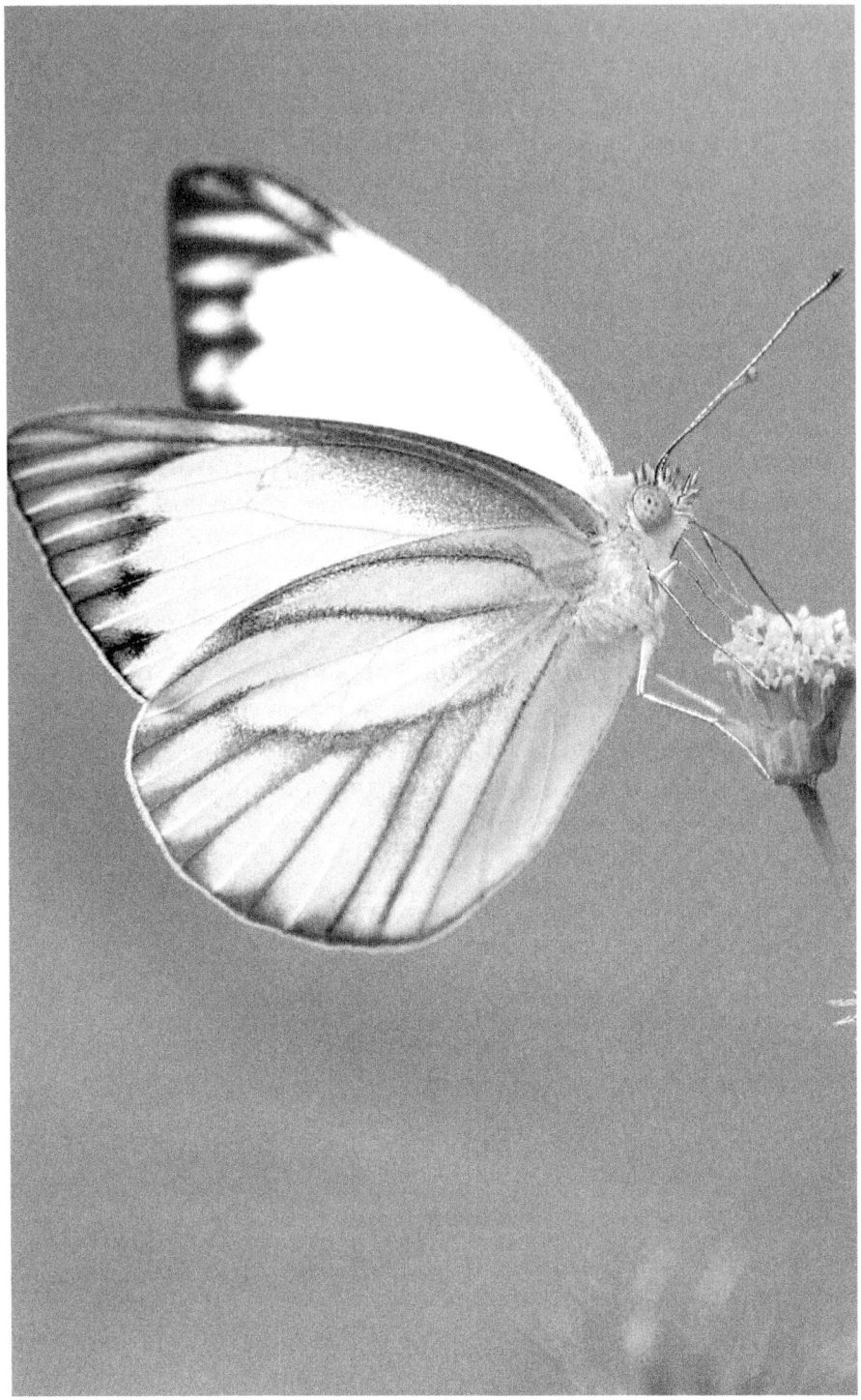

CHAPTER 8: RENEWAL AND TRANSFORMATION – REBUILDING HEALTH AND LIFE

Having journeyed from late-stage cancer to recovery, I have come to cherish life more deeply, gaining a profound understanding of its fragility and resilience. This extraordinary experience not only reignited my passion for living but also restored my unwavering confidence in the future. Regaining my health brought about a profound shift in my outlook on life and the world, allowing me to embrace life anew with a fresh perspective.

In this chapter, I will share my experiences of reshaping my life after recovery and the profound insights and wisdom gained from this journey. Overcoming cancer was not the end of the story but the beginning of a new chapter—a gateway to the holistic transformation of both my mind and life. Although this journey was fraught with pain and challenges, it gifted me invaluable wisdom and a deeper understanding of existence.

It is often only when one approaches the edge of mortality that a true awakening occurs, revealing the profound meaning of life. This experience taught me to treasure and express gratitude for every moment of being alive. Through reflecting on life and cultivating inner awareness, I found an unprecedented sense of fulfillment, one no longer reliant on external success or fleeting happiness. I learned to infuse love and kindness into every ordinary moment, experiencing a sense of inner peace and joy.

The path to recovery extended beyond physical healing—it required the emotional and social reintegration of life. I needed to confront changes that had been ignored or set aside, embarking on a journey of rediscovering life and cultivating wisdom through inner resilience. As I gradually returned to normalcy, the fears that had shadowed me during treatment began to dissipate, replaced by a deeper understanding of life's essence. Those darkest moments, paradoxically, became a source of strength for my future.

This experience profoundly transformed my mindset. In the past, I pursued many things with relentless determination and anxiety, yet now, their significance has shifted dramatically. Conquering cancer led me to reevaluate my life's priorities and redefine the true meaning of happiness and success. Through reflecting on life's core values, my perspective has broadened, and my priorities have been realigned.

Today, I have embarked on an entirely new chapter of life. With a more composed and open heart, I face each new day, ready to embrace the future with clarity and resilience.

The Essence of Rebuilding Life

In the process of reshaping my life, I have learned to face challenges with a more balanced and thoughtful approach. Reintegrating into daily work and social life was not my sole objective. The true essence lay in rediscovering inner peace and fulfillment through the everyday experiences of life. This awakening has filled me with gratitude for life and enabled me to adapt better to the coexistence with my new post-cancer reality. I am no longer merely a survivor of illness; instead, I have found a renewed self, rebuilt with wisdom and balance. Now, no matter how chaotic the world may be or what events life may bring, I can find a haven of tranquility and peace within myself.

Embracing The Preciousness Of Life

Having endured the trials of cancer, I now have a renewed perspective on the passage of time. My lifestyle and character have undergone significant changes. In the past, my understanding of life was superficial, but now I hold a profound reverence for its brevity and fragility. I no longer fixate on fleeting and surface-level accomplishments; instead, I cherish each moment of life, immersing myself in and appreciating what truly matters—health, family, and inner peace.

The everyday moments I once took for granted or overlooked—like breathing, walking, sharing warm moments with family, or even the sound of birdsong—now feel extraordinarily precious and worthy of deep appreciation. Every past experience has left an indelible mark on my heart, shaping the person I am today and enriching my current life with profound meaning. Reflecting on life's beauty, I am reminded that simply being alive is an incomparably precious gift. I can tangibly feel my life reviving and flourishing once again.

I vividly recall the day when the doctor informed me that I might only have six months to live. The helplessness I felt then remains etched in my memory, as vivid as if it happened yesterday. Now, ten years later, I am still living a healthy and grateful life, savoring every moment. That dark period taught me resilience and gave me a deeper understanding of the true meaning of life. From standing at the brink of death to living a full and healthy life today, I have gained a renewed appreciation and a profound sense of gratitude for existence.

Redefining Life's Priorities

After enduring the arduous battle with illness, I have profoundly reconsidered and restructured my life's priorities. There was a time when professional achievements, financial success, and social status consumed nearly all my focus. I once believed that success stemmed from external validation. However, after facing the brink of life and death, these pursuits have gradually faded from my view. Life has imparted a profound lesson: true happiness does not lie in outward accomplishments but in inner peace, the warmth of family, and a deep connection with the world.

Returning To Family And Building A Sanctuary

On this journey of rebirth, family has gradually become the center of my life. During my recovery, I dedicated significant time and effort not only to fighting cancer but also to fulfilling a long-held dream of building a home. Remarkably, these two endeavors brought rewards almost simultaneously: as the house was completed, my health also began to miraculously improve. This house is more than just a residence; it is a sanctuary in a chaotic world. During those darkest days, the process of building the house became a source of hope and solace for me. Every beam, every wall, and every structure represented my perseverance and determination, and its completion symbolized my renewal.

I have come to understand that time spent with family is invaluable. In the past, my pursuit of career goals often made me overlook the precious moments shared with loved ones. Now, every moment is irreplaceable. Whether it's a simple family dinner or an evening walk under the setting sun, these ordinary moments have become the most significant part of my life. My home has become the warmest harbor for my soul, a place of refuge and belonging no matter how fierce the storms outside.

Rediscovering The Beauty Of Life

Each morning, as the first rays of sunlight pour into the room, illuminating every corner in golden light, I feel a profound sense of gratitude. The tranquil beauty outside the window fills my heart with peace, joy, and contentment. To me, this is more than just the start of a new day—it is a divine gift, granting me another chance to experience the beauty of life. The fresh air feels almost tangible, and this house has come to symbolize my rebirth. Watching my son grow, step into society, and secure an ideal internship fills me with immense pride and fulfillment.

By redefining my life's priorities, I have not only discovered what truly matters but also learned to shift my focus from chasing external achievements to cherishing every small moment of life. Those once-overlooked details now hold a central place in my daily existence, and I have cultivated a heart full of gratitude for everything. This illness also brought a deeper awareness of the critical importance of health—it is not only the foundation of all future dreams and goals but also the cornerstone of my present life. Today, success is no longer defined by external standards but by inner peace and contentment. Through this shift in mindset, I have rediscovered a profound connection with the essence of life itself.

Strengthening Psychological Resilience and Emotional Power

The challenges of cancer instilled in me a level of emotional maturity

I had never experienced before. Over time, I became more resilient, learned techniques for emotional regulation, and discovered ways to maintain inner peace and tranquility in the face of fear. This sense of calm gradually became the cornerstone of my life; whenever I encountered new challenges, I was able to remain composed and determined, growing step by step into a stronger version of myself.

Although cancer forced me to confront mortality, it also gave me the opportunity to reexamine the meaning of life. I learned to let go of excessive worries about the future and to cherish every authentic moment. Each day became more precious than ever because I understood that the clarity and contentment I now experienced were things my former self had never truly appreciated.

Life is inherently full of uncertainties, and many things are beyond my control. While external circumstances cannot always be changed, I found that by adjusting my mindset or approaching situations from a different perspective, I could often achieve unexpectedly positive results. This shift in attitude has enabled me to find motivation even in adversity. Whatever challenges I face, I am now able to see the positive and bright side of situations. This optimism continues to shape my unyielding psychological resilience.

When difficulties arise again, I no longer react with fear or anxiety as I once did. Instead, I focus on small progress and derive a sense of accomplishment from every step of persistence and growth. Whether it's in daily routines or significant events, I handle situations with poise and confidence. Even the smallest victories bring me deep joy, gratitude, and fulfillment.

More importantly, this experience has taught me that vulnerability is not shameful. Accepting my imperfections and seeking help from others when necessary has not made me feel weak; instead, it has revealed the profound warmth of human connection. Sharing my feelings and accepting the support and encouragement of others has provided me with unparalleled emotional comfort and confidence. These emotional supports have allowed me to remain steadfast in the face of difficulties. They have given me the courage to move forward and helped me realize that true resilience is born of mutual care and understanding. This kind of support makes us all stronger.

This inner growth and accumulation have allowed me to face life's ups and downs with greater composure. Even in moments of despair, I can find the confidence to rise again and emerge from each setback with renewed strength to face the challenges ahead.

Rebuilding a Healthy Lifestyle

Today, my commitment to health has reached an unprecedented level. In the past, I often overlooked the importance of a healthy lifestyle, assuming that as long as life was going well, there was no need to pay special attention to my body. However, this experience has taught me that health is not a given—it requires consistent effort and meticulous care. Health has become the core of my daily life, not just an option but a steadfast commitment and attitude toward life.

In terms of diet, I now prioritize balanced nutrition, ensuring my body receives comprehensive support. Eating is no longer a matter of convenience but a thoughtfully curated process to maintain and promote long-term health. I have also come to deeply appreciate the indispensable value of regular exercise, which has become a fundamental pillar for sustaining physical strength and vitality. Moreover, I have successfully eliminated unhealthy habits such as irregular schedules, poor dietary preferences, and smoking.

As my health gradually improved, these changes have made me stronger than ever, significantly enhancing my quality of life and work efficiency. These adjustments not only brought physical benefits but also profoundly altered the trajectory of my life. At the same time, they fostered a positive mindset, enabling me to handle life's challenges and minor inconveniences with greater ease. More importantly, these healthy habits have become the foundation of my personal growth, infusing me with enduring physical and mental vitality and an optimistic outlook on life. They not only safeguard my physical well-being but also imbue my life with new meaning and direction, allowing me to find fulfillment and richness in every ordinary day.

Strengthening Family and Social Bonds

Emotional support has been like a lighthouse in the darkness, guiding my way and providing warmth during the loneliest moments. After my recovery, I reexamined human connections, realizing the profound importance of family and relationships in life. Whereas I once prioritized personal career and achievements, I now actively nurture these invaluable relationships, showing greater care for my loved ones' lives and sharing our mutual feelings. These emotional connections have become the most solid pillars of my existence. Whether it's the warmth of family interactions or meaningful conversations with friends, these bonds now hold an irreplaceable position in my life, providing enduring emotional support and comfort.

Each family gathering, every phone call from a friend, and even a simple greeting from someone reminds me of the crucial role these relationships play in my life. They are not just companions; they are my source of motivation. No matter the challenges or joys that lie ahead, these precious bonds will continue to provide strength. Together, we will always stand side by side, serving as each other's steadfast support and refuge.

This journey through illness has taught me to cherish every relationship more deeply, revealing that these connections go far beyond everyday interactions. Family, friendships, and social networks have not only provided emotional solace but also offered irreplaceable support and a drive for renewal during my most challenging times. The significance of these relationships brings balance and security to my inner world while granting me a deeper sense of fulfillment and purpose in life.

Grateful and Giving Back to Life

Experiencing life and death has taught me the fragility and preciousness of existence. It has made me realize that every ordinary day is worthy of respect and gratitude. After recovering physically, my sense of appreciation for life has deepened profoundly. I no longer allow myself to be troubled by trivial matters but focus instead on what truly matters. This experience has made me more humble and has awakened in me an undeniable responsibility to share my cancer journey and help others. I have proactively begun telling my story, hoping to bring hope and strength to those facing similar struggles. I firmly believe that through sharing, I can help others find the courage to move forward, guiding them out of the shadows of despair and into the light of life.

Life is fleeting, and waking up each morning with energy is a priceless gift. Facing life with a heart full of gratitude has become my best approach to handling challenges. This gratitude goes beyond internal emotions; it has transformed into tangible actions. I have come to realize that helping others provides rewards far greater than I could have imagined. Whether it's patiently listening to their stories or offering practical support when needed, the act of helping others has not only enriched my own life but has also given me a deeper understanding of life's true meaning.

I now understand that genuine gratitude does not stop at feelings of thankfulness but extends to concrete actions that give back to life and create meaningful value and fulfilling experiences. Even the smallest act of kindness—a warm smile or a sincere word of encouragement—can ripple through someone's heart and bring unexpected change. With this spirit of gratitude, I continue walking the path of helping others heal, striving to help more people find hope in despair, reignite their faith in life, and connect with the powerful force of existence.

This gratitude has not only brought profound personal growth but has also deepened my appreciation for the beauty and value of human connections and support. With this belief, I am committed to brightening others' lives with care and compassion, bringing warmth to those in difficult times, and being a source of comfort and support when they are at their lowest. I aim to help them rediscover their inner strength and once again feel the warmth and kindness of life. This is not only my way of giving back to life with gratitude but also a solemn promise to live with love and resilience. I will continue forward, carrying the light of hope to those who need it most.

Spiritual Growth and Inner Reflection

Cancer not only gave me a second chance at physical life but also led to a profound transformation on a spiritual level. This journey compelled me to continuously reflect on the true meaning and purpose of life, helping me cultivate a deeper connection with my inner self. I discovered within me a profound sense of tranquility that allows me to face life's challenges with composure and draw valuable lessons from them, turning each experience into a catalyst for personal growth and spiritual awakening.

In the past, I viewed life's events as mere coincidences. Now, I firmly believe in the deep interconnection of all things within the universe. Each moment and every experience is no longer isolated; together, they form the complete journey of my inner growth, spiritual transformation, and awakening. This has enriched my spiritual world, deepened my understanding of life, and revealed the unique meaning behind every trial. This realization has enabled me to accept life's ups and downs with equanimity, fostering a deeper understanding of myself and my connection to the world and even the greater dimensions of the universe.

This turning point in my destiny, though arduous, has brought me through this phase not only with restored health and a renewed sense of life but also with profound wisdom and insight. It has allowed me to reevaluate life and view all things in the world from a fresh perspective. Every experience holds significance, guiding me step by step toward a more authentic and complete version of myself. Often, when a person feels they have reached a dead end, life unexpectedly reveals a path filled with opportunities and possibilities. Holding steadfast to this belief provides us with the strength to rise again from the depths and empowers us to stand taller and see further.

Self-Acceptance

Learning to accept oneself and letting go of harsh self-judgment is essential to connecting with inner strength. Self-acceptance involves treating yourself with kindness and cultivating self-compassion, fostering a lasting sense of balance and security within. Even in the face of difficulties and adversity, this foundation allows you to draw strength from within. After undergoing this transformative journey, I gradually learned to embrace the uncertainties of life and to release the need to control what is beyond my reach. I no longer feel anxious about the unknown future but have instead found ways to anchor myself in the present, cultivating a sense of peace and serenity.

Although I have been cancer-free for years, I deeply understand that the only constant in life is change. Many things may not unfold as expected or turn out as desired. The future will likely hold new, unpredictable challenges, but I have learned to accept and adapt to life's impermanence. I now view life's ups and downs with calmness, recognizing them as steps in my personal growth. Reflecting on the past, those struggles and moments of despair that once seemed insurmountable have become invaluable experiences that shaped who I am today. The initial diagnosis once filled me with hopelessness, yet it ultimately became the start of a new chapter, guiding me toward a renewed journey of life. That dark period brought not only physical recovery but also taught me to slow down and savor every detail of life, even amidst the storm.

This trial brought profound reflection and growth, granting me an unprecedented sense of inner peace and wisdom. I have come to realize that every moment is precious, and when we learn to draw strength from these moments, we discover a clarity and resilience within ourselves. Today, I face each day with a positive mindset, knowing that no matter the challenges I encounter, my inner strength will sustain me. With gratitude and determination, I embrace every new beginning that life has to offer.

A New Definition of Career

and Personal Growth

The experience of battling cancer not only altered my perspective on life but also led me to reassess the meaning of my career. This challenging journey acted as a mirror, reflecting how my obsession with work had once consumed other aspects of my life. My career had previously been my everything, and I viewed professional achievements as the sole measure of my self-worth. Each accomplishment, each recognition in the workplace, drove me relentlessly forward, as if it were the only validation of my existence. However, as my health gradually recovered, I began to see with increasing clarity that true happiness does not stem from external achievements but from inner contentment and a harmonious balance in life.

This experience not only compelled me to redefine the meaning of my career but also propelled profound growth and transformation within. I no longer see my career as the centerpiece of my life; instead, I have learned to find a healthy balance between work and personal life. I have become a new version of myself—someone who treasures everyday moments and has a broader perspective that extends beyond work. Today, while my career remains an important part of my life, it is no longer my sole focus. I now contemplate how my career can contribute to my growth and bring me inner fulfillment, rather than merely chasing professional accolades and status. Achievements in the workplace are still meaningful, but they no longer define my entirety. I have come to understand that work should not consume all my time and energy but should instead serve as a vehicle for achieving personal goals and enriching my life experiences.

In this process, I have grown more resolute and composed. I have learned how to manage work-related stress and discovered a rhythm that suits me. Whatever storms my future career may bring, I am prepared to face them with a calm and confident attitude. Even if the future holds unknowns or severe life challenges, I know I can maintain an inner peace and acceptance, accompanied by a profound sense of tranquility and strength.

Thus, regardless of the successes I may achieve in my career, I remain clear that this is only one part of my life, not its entirety. By redefining the role of my career, I have gained a deeper inner strength, enabling me to face any challenges life may present without fear. This rebirth has illuminated the true value of life, leaving my heart stronger and more serene. I no longer fear the unknown but have learned to draw strength from faith, hope, and love as I stride confidently toward the future.

Conclusion

This chapter reflects on the new life I embraced after overcoming cancer and the profound lessons it imparted. It is only after emerging from the depths of despair that one can truly appreciate the brilliance of the sunlight. These difficult moments taught me that perseverance ultimately leads to light. Life's ups and downs are inevitable, but every hardship brings growth and insight. As long as we do not give up, hope will always be waiting on the horizon. I continue to move forward with resilience, growing each day, and cherishing the love and support of those around me, which has made life more beautiful than ever.

Having gone through this journey, I have developed the habit of regular self-reflection. This practice serves as an excellent way to understand myself, enabling me to continually discover my inner potential and sources of strength. I have come to realize that life is meant to be experienced, not lived in pursuit of unattainable perfection. Because of this, I no longer demand a flawless existence but have learned to calmly accept the changes I cannot control.

I treasure and give thanks for every moment, allowing each day the possibility of being the most beautiful one yet. Whatever the future holds, I will face it with gratitude, inner strength, and wisdom, growing with each experience and pressing forward with determination. Gratitude is not just an attitude but a powerful form of emotional healing, allowing me to remain steadfast and clear-headed in the face of life's challenges.

Healing is not simply about recovering from illness but about rebuilding balance and harmony in both mind and body. This experience has made me stronger and shaped who I am today. This journey has deepened my understanding of life's meaning and taught me to approach each day with an open and resilient heart. It is the inner strength and the power of belief that enable me to create positive life experiences and take control of my destiny.

To conclude this chapter, I turn to the famous words of Friedrich Nietzsche, the German philosopher, literary critic, poet, and cultural critic (1844–1900): "That which does not kill me makes me stronger." I hope this timeless quote inspires you, as it reflects Nietzsche's profound insight into adversity and human potential. May it encourage all of us to grow through challenges and courageously achieve breakthroughs in life.

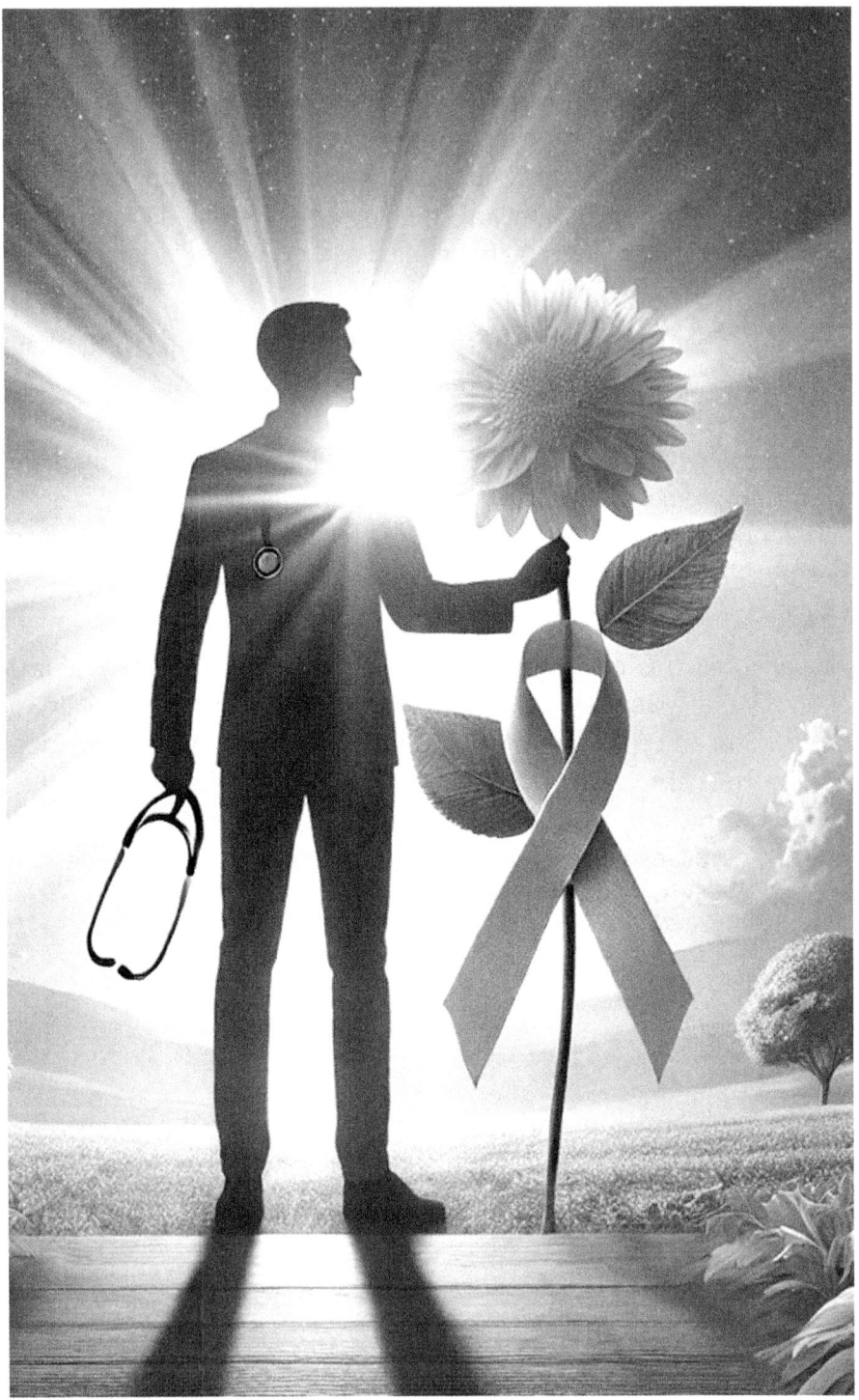

CHAPTER 9: UNWAVERING BELIEF – HOPE FOR RECOVERY AND A VISION FOR THE FUTURE

This chapter aims to provide inspiration and support to those navigating similar challenges, offering them renewed courage and confidence. Although cancer has long been regarded as one of the most formidable diseases in the medical field, advancements in medicine have led many countries to begin treating cancer as a manageable chronic condition.

Through my own journey of battling cancer and helping others overcome it, I have become increasingly convinced that cancer can be defeated. The key lies in finding the recovery methods that work best for each individual while simultaneously adjusting one's mindset and strategies for coping. For me, cancer was not just a physical struggle but also a profound test of both mind and body. Strengthening oneself and fortifying one's inner resolve are essential to withstanding the pressures and challenges that arise throughout this journey.

My victory over cancer is not only a personal achievement but also a testament to the progress of modern medicine. Finding the right recovery approach is critical, and my experience has allowed me to witness firsthand the incredible self-healing capabilities of the human body. This realization has prompted me to reexamine and transcend traditional understandings of cancer. Over the years, I have not only achieved full recovery but also emerged healthier than before my diagnosis, with a renewed perspective and a deeper appreciation for life.

For this reason, I hope to share my story to help others, particularly those who are in the midst of hardship. No matter the medical prognosis, no matter how daunting the situation may seem—even in moments that appear utterly hopeless—it is vital to maintain an unwavering belief in oneself and the body's extraordinary capacity for recovery.

From Despair to Hope: A True Testament of Success

When the doctor informed me of the severity of my condition and the grim prognosis, I faced not only physical suffering but also the uncertainty of the future and immense emotional stress. At that moment, I felt as though I had been plunged into endless darkness, with the illness appearing insurmountable. However, despite the waves of fear and confusion that often engulfed me, I chose not to surrender to fate but to actively seek out every possible avenue for recovery.

I quickly realized that passively waiting would do nothing to change my situation. I resolved to fight for every possible chance at recovery. As discussed in Chapter 3 of this book, the first step was to gain a thorough understanding of my illness and master every detail about cancer and potential recovery methods. During countless sleepless nights, I pored over medical literature, kept up with the latest research advancements, and took charge of my recovery journey. I engaged with experts from various fields, asked specific questions, and sought tailored recovery strategies. Through this process of self-education and exploration, I came to see that cancer is not invincible. Advances in modern medicine have provided unprecedented opportunities for recovery, and combining alternative therapies with holistic healing approaches offers immense potential.

Through this journey, I evolved from a helpless individual affected by cancer into a proactive steward of my own health, regaining control over my life. By consistently learning and researching, I discovered numerous innovative therapies that have brought hope to many battling cancer. I combined these new approaches with traditional recovery methods, as detailed in Chapter 5. This integrative recovery strategy enabled me to effectively address various challenges, restore balance and vitality to my body, and ultimately achieve full recovery.

The turning point in my recovery came during the mid-stages of my battle with cancer. At that time, my body had been pushed to its limits, and the side effects nearly drained me of the courage to continue. Yet, just when I felt powerless, my body began to respond positively, and the effects of recovery became increasingly evident. I could clearly sense improvement; cancer was no longer an undefeatable adversary but a challenge that could be overcome.

This experience solidified my belief that everyone possesses the strength to overcome illness. The key lies in changing our perception of cancer and finding recovery methods that suit our individual needs. By harnessing both physical and psychological resources, maintaining a positive mindset and unwavering determination, and drawing on multifaceted support, we can transform these internal reserves into tangible recovery outcomes.

As I reflected in Chapter 7, alongside medical support, spiritual and emotional strength are equally indispensable. A positive attitude and firm belief are irreplaceable pillars in the fight against cancer. Ultimately, it was the combined forces of physical, emotional, and social support that helped me emerge from adversity.

Now, though I have fully recovered, I remain committed to helping others and supporting them as they regain control of their lives. This journey has taught me how to take ownership of my health and shown me that cancer is not the end of life. Instead, it is a new beginning—a chance to rebuild oneself and emerge stronger and more resilient than ever before.

Passing On Strength: Helping Others Heal

In the preface and throughout other chapters of this book, we have mentioned Julia multiple times, but we have yet to share her story in detail. Now, let us delve into her courageous and hopeful journey, recounting how she tenaciously overcame cancer. Julia's story is a poignant testament to the resilience and strength of the human spirit, serving as a powerful reminder of the unyielding fight for life.

After my recovery, I sought to help others battling cancer in various ways, and Julia's story stands out as one of the most moving and inspiring. In February 2023, Julia was diagnosed with advanced pancreatic cancer and lung cancer. Both of these cancers are notoriously challenging to treat, especially when diagnosed in their later stages, as symptoms often remain hidden until surgical options are no longer viable. Pancreatic cancer, in particular, is known as the "king of cancers" due to its high mortality rate and rapid progression, leaving few medical interventions available. Julia's diagnosis came with a devastating prognosis: a life expectancy of just three to six months.

The news hit like a bolt of lightning, shattering Julia and her family's world, leaving them little time to process or prepare. Following the diagnosis, Julia, her family, and her friends quickly began gathering information, scouring every available resource on these cancers in search of possible treatments. Yet, the more they learned, the more their hope dimmed. The literature painted a grim picture, especially regarding late-stage pancreatic cancer. Confronted with such overwhelming odds, Julia felt utterly helpless, burdened by excruciating physical pain and immense psychological trauma. While undergoing extensive medical examinations, she began putting her affairs in order—planning her estate, managing her bank accounts, dividing family assets, and even making funeral arrangements to prepare for the worst.

Despite the immense physical and emotional strain, with my encouragement and support, Julia resolved not to give up. She began undergoing a combination of chemotherapy and immunotherapy. Although these treatments came with severe side effects that left her physically drained and emotionally volatile, she remained steadfast. In addition, she explored alternative therapies mentioned in Chapter 5, embracing them as a last resort and a glimmer of hope. Her emotional journey was akin to a rollercoaster—fluctuating between moments of hope and despair. Witnessing her struggles resonated deeply with me, as I had endured similar emotional turmoil during my own battle, though Julia's circumstances were even more dire.

Remarkably, Julia's survival far exceeded the doctors' initial predictions, culminating in what can only be described as a medical miracle. By July 2024, routine PET and CT scans revealed an astonishing outcome: cancer cells in both her pancreas and lungs had nearly disappeared, leaving only a 5-millimeter scar with no active disease.

This extraordinary progress left not only her family and friends in disbelief but also her medical team, who hailed it as an incredible achievement. Julia's recovery was nothing short of a miraculous reversal, turning an unattainable dream into reality. It brought immeasurable joy and deep emotional relief to everyone involved. Her recovery was not only a breakthrough in medical terms but also a profound spiritual triumph, offering solace as if she had narrowly escaped the clutches of death. This transformation reinvigorated all those who stood by her side, reaffirming the power of perseverance and the eternal light of hope.

Despite this unprecedented success, Julia struggled to fully embrace the miraculous turn of events. I found myself torn between understanding her emotions and grappling with my own questions about her hesitancy. After much reflection, I realized that her subconscious mind might not yet be ready to accept this sudden deliverance from such a harrowing ordeal. Her response, initially perplexing, began to make sense: the profound emotional scars left by the diagnosis and its associated trauma could not heal overnight. It became clear that the psychological healing from such a life-altering journey requires its own time and space.

Julia's diagnosis of two deadly cancers and the knowledge of her limited life expectancy left indelible marks on her psyche. Although her body has healed, her soul continues to need time to process and adapt to this unimaginable reversal of fortune. Her story stands as a testament not only to the miraculous potential of recovery but also to the enduring resilience required to heal both body and spirit.

Here are some possible explanations, which may stem from psychological and emotional factors:

1. Trauma and Psychological Distress

Her severe illness brought about a profoundly traumatic experience. Even though her condition has improved, she may still be living in a state of persistent fear and caution. Trauma often leaves a psychological "imprint," making it difficult for her to fully accept or believe that she can achieve complete recovery.

2. Loss of Confidence in Her Body

The severity of her illness likely undermined her confidence in her own body. Given the advanced stage of two cancers, it may be challenging for her to believe that her body can regain its strength and health. Even with evident improvements, her trust in her physical well-being remains fragile.

3. Fear of Recurrence

Fear of recurrence is particularly common among cancer survivors. This deeply ingrained "fear of recurrence" may prevent her from fully embracing the idea of recovery. Instead, she may remain in a state of vigilance and doubt, psychologically preparing herself for the possibility of future relapses or complications.

4. Psychological Dependence

Some individuals may develop a psychological dependence on their illness, becoming accustomed to its presence. Even when their condition improves, they may subconsciously struggle to accept this reality, finding it difficult to detach from the role of being unwell.

5. Identity Transformation

Chronic illness can significantly alter one's self-image. For many, the emotional association with their illness becomes part of their identity, making it hard to accept a "healthy" self. For her, the illness may have become an intrinsic part of her identity, making the transition to post-recovery life emotionally challenging.

6. Existential and Spiritual Confusion

Severe illness often prompts existential questions and reshapes one's understanding of self and life. She may subconsciously attach profound meaning or messages to her illness, leading to internal conflict when embracing a "healthy" state.

7. Cognitive Distortions

In some cases, individuals develop distorted perceptions of their illness, such as the belief that "my illness is incurable." Even after recovery, such deeply ingrained beliefs are difficult to reverse quickly, creating barriers to accepting their improved condition. This could be a residual effect of the earlier trauma and psychological distress.

The interplay of these factors may have collectively contributed to her psychological state. I firmly believe that, over time, Julia will gradually overcome the lingering shadows and profound trauma of her past and find a path toward inner light. I will continue to visit her or speak with her regularly, providing ongoing emotional support and closely monitoring her recovery progress. Julia's story is yet another miracle I have witnessed firsthand, reaffirming the possibility of recovery from cancer. Her resilience and perseverance fill me with immense pride and comfort. I am convinced that as the years pass, the wounds of her soul will gradually heal, and life will open a new, warm chapter for her, bringing peace and solace.

Julia's experience is not merely a tale of triumph over cancer; it is a profound testament to hope, faith, and persistence. Even in the face of the harshest realities, miracles can occur in the most unexpected moments. This has strengthened my belief that as long as we do not give up, there is always a glimmer of light awaiting us.

Thus, when confronting cancer, it is crucial to choose effective recovery strategies promptly. As demonstrated by both my journey and Julia's story, returning to a path of health is entirely possible, even in advanced stages. When we believe in ourselves and the power of nature, opportunities for transformation will arise.

Julia's return to health has deeply shown me that in critical moments of life, meeting the right person at the right time can fundamentally change one's destiny. Leo Martin's presence was like a warm light illuminating Julia's life during her darkest and most desperate times. His encouragement and support reignited Julia's hope for life and strengthened her determination to keep fighting.

In life, encountering someone who extends a helping hand in times of greatest need is extraordinarily rare and something to be profoundly grateful for. Leo was undoubtedly a pivotal figure in Julia's life. In Chinese culture, the term "guiren" is often used to describe those who selflessly offer help, support, or guidance during critical moments of adversity, decision-making, or life transitions. Such individuals are regarded as key players in one's destiny, often having a positive and decisive influence on a person's life or career. This assistance goes beyond material support to include emotional encouragement and the provision of pivotal opportunities.

Therefore, Leo is not only the most important person in Julia's life but also a guiding light in her destiny. He led her out of the darkness, bringing her hope and courage. Because of his presence, Julia's life trajectory was completely transformed, allowing her to be reborn and embrace a life filled with hope.

Witnessing how she rose from the depths of despair, bravely facing the challenges of cancer and surmounting each obstacle, I am deeply convinced of the power of love and support to transcend all difficulties. No matter how cruel fate may be, as long as there is warmth in companionship and genuine trust, light and new opportunities will always be waiting ahead.

Hope for Healing Belongs to Everyone

Through my personal experiences and the support I've provided to others on their successful journeys against cancer, I have gained a deeper understanding of physical recovery. In this process, I not only acquired valuable insights into the nature of illnesses but also recognized that the journey to healing is unique to each individual. As Hildegard von Bingen (1098–1179), the renowned medieval German composer, writer, and natural scientist, once said: "Every illness has the potential to be healed, but not every person can recover." This statement highlights the complexity of dealing with illness and underscores the importance of individual differences.

Theoretically, most illnesses possess the potential for recovery. The human body has remarkable self-healing capabilities, and the onset of disease is often the result of multiple interacting factors, such as lifestyle, mental state, genetic predispositions, and more. These factors significantly influence the development and progression of illness and play a critical role in the recovery process, as discussed in earlier chapters. Furthermore, certain spiritual traditions suggest that diseases symbolize imbalances in the body's energy or represent inner challenges that humans must confront. These perspectives profoundly shape how people understand health and approach illness.

Despite Advances in Modern Medicine, Some Diseases Remain Uncured. The reasons behind the incomplete cure of certain diseases can be attributed to the following factors:

1. Lifestyle Habits

Unhealthy lifestyles and excessive stress gradually weaken the body's immune system and even impact recovery outcomes. If these habits are not addressed during treatment, the chances of recovery are significantly reduced.

2. Individual Differences

Responses to interventions vary from person to person, influenced by factors such as genetics, physical constitution, and overall health. The same treatment plan may yield vastly different results across individuals. As such, personalized recovery plans often lead to more favorable outcomes.

3. Disease Progression

Delays in early detection and intervention, slow individual responses to adjustments, or missed opportunities due to misdiagnosis can make late-stage recovery efforts significantly more challenging, reducing the likelihood of a cure.

4. Complexity of the Disease

Certain diseases are inherently complex, often involving damage to multiple systems or organs. The absence of effective treatment options can further complicate the recovery process.

5. Recurrence of Illness

Some diseases recur due to insufficiently scientific treatment approaches, inadequate individual treatment strategies, or unhealthy lifestyles. These recurrences increase the difficulty of achieving a full recovery.

6. Accessibility of Medical Interventions

Economic disparities and unequal access to medical resources prevent some individuals from receiving timely and effective treatment. This inequitable distribution of healthcare not only impacts the likelihood of a cure but also delays diagnosis and treatment, further diminishing recovery prospects.

7. Psychological State and Motivation

Psychological well-being and the will to recover play critical roles in the treatment process. A lack of psychological support or sufficient motivation for recovery can hinder the effectiveness of even the most advanced medical strategies. Strong psychological support can boost confidence and foster a positive physiological response to recovery, facilitating the healing process. Therefore, integrating medical technology with mental health support is essential for a successful recovery.

8. Lack of Discipline and Commitment

Maintaining a healthy lifestyle requires long-term discipline, and the absence of this consistency often leads to disease recurrence, complicating the path to a cure.

Traditional treatments such as surgery, radiation, and chemotherapy remain the primary approaches for managing and eradicating cancer. However, as cancer cells mutate and spread, medical interventions become increasingly complex. A deeper understanding of cancer and a more comprehensive, systematic approach to recovery are crucial.

By thoroughly understanding the underlying causes and progression of diseases, while respecting individual differences and prioritizing overall health maintenance, everyone has the potential to regain wellness. The key lies in identifying the recovery path that best suits the individual. Regardless of the disease faced, a positive mindset, unwavering belief, personalized recovery plans, and scientifically sound medical interventions are essential and indispensable pillars for overcoming illness and restoring health.

Medical Breakthroughs:

A New Era and Dawn of Healing

In recent years, approaches to the diagnosis and treatment of cancer have undergone profound transformations. With the rapid advancement of science and technology, cancer management has entered a new era, making the complete cure of cancer an increasingly tangible reality. Whether at the early stages of diagnosis or facing advanced stages of the disease, no one should abandon hope or miss the opportunity for recovery. Over the past decades, significant breakthroughs in cancer research have not only greatly improved recovery outcomes but also reshaped many traditional perceptions of the disease.

Today, modern medicine has enabled cancer treatments to become more precise, effectively targeting cancer cells while minimizing damage to healthy tissues. This progress has significantly reduced the side effects of traditional therapies, thereby improving the quality of life during recovery. At the same time, scientists continue to explore ways to enhance the immune system's ability to identify and eliminate cancer cells more effectively. As a result, cancer is no longer seen as an insurmountable challenge but as a disease that can be managed, recovered from, and potentially eradicated.

In recent years, the widespread adoption of emerging recovery methods has not only substantially increased survival rates for cancer patients but has also brought renewed hope to those who could not be cured through traditional approaches. Personalized recovery plans, tailored to individual needs, have replaced the outdated "one-size-fits-all" strategy, achieving greater effectiveness in the recovery process.

Simultaneously, innovations in early cancer detection technologies have continued to evolve. Advanced diagnostic tools now allow for the identification of cancer at earlier stages, enabling timely intervention. This significantly reduces the risk of cancer progression and greatly enhances the likelihood of successful recovery. The importance of early detection and intervention has been increasingly validated by research, offering cancer-affected individuals more opportunities to regain their health.

The rapid progress in medical science has not only made cancer interventions more efficient and precise but has also provided invaluable hope to individuals with cancer and their families. Today, cancer management strategies are no longer solely focused on extending life but are advancing toward achieving complete health.

Therefore, whether newly diagnosed or in advanced stages of the disease, individuals should embrace the recovery opportunities brought about by scientific progress and actively seek personalized recovery strategies. The future of cancer recovery lies not merely in "survival" but in "healing" and improving "quality of life."

Next, we will explore several modern cancer support strategies and groundbreaking medical innovations that have demonstrated significant potential in the cancer recovery process.

Modern Approaches To Cancer Management: Advances And Prospects

From immunotherapy, gene editing, and precision medicine to liquid biopsies and early detection technologies, these cutting-edge advancements have brought new hope to cancer-affected individuals worldwide, making the goal of defeating cancer increasingly achievable.

Below are several representative modern support strategies:

1. Radiation Therapy
Utilizes high-energy radiation to destroy cancer cells and reduce tumor spread.

2. Chemotherapy
Employs drugs to kill or slow the growth of cancer cells, commonly used for various types of cancer.

3. Immunotherapy
Activates the body's immune system to identify and eliminate cancer cells, particularly effective for individuals unresponsive to traditional treatments.

4. Precision Medicine
Develops personalized plans based on an individual's genetic profile, precisely targeting the specific characteristics of tumors.

5. Hormone Therapy
Regulates hormone levels to treat certain cancers, particularly effective for hormone-related cancers.

6. Targeted Therapy
Focuses on specific molecules within cancer cells, minimizing harm to healthy cells.

The progress of these modern recovery strategies has not only opened new possibilities for cancer management but also provided substantial support to individuals worldwide engaged in the fight against cancer.

The Innovative Revolution In Cancer Management

The field of cancer recovery is entering an unprecedented era of innovation. The integration of artificial intelligence, genetic science, and nanomedicine is not only transforming how we approach cancer but also providing cancer-affected individuals with more personalized and precise recovery options.

Cutting-Edge Innovations in Cancer Treatment – Here are some key breakthroughs:

1. Artificial Intelligence (AI)

AI has played a pivotal role in the early detection of cancer. By rapidly analyzing vast amounts of imaging data, it significantly improves diagnostic accuracy and efficiency, enabling doctors to identify cancer earlier and develop targeted strategies. This technology accelerates the diagnostic process, reduces the likelihood of misdiagnosis, and grants cancer patients invaluable time for recovery.

2. Genetic Testing

Advances in genetic science allow individuals with a family history of cancer to undergo more precise risk assessments and design personalized prevention strategies. Genetic testing enables the early identification of cancer risks, facilitating earlier intervention and prevention.

3. Metabolic Therapy

Metabolic therapy targets cancer cell growth by disrupting their metabolism, aiming to halt the spread of cancer cells without harming healthy ones. This precision-focused approach minimizes collateral damage while effectively managing cancer progression.

4. Nanomedicine

The application of nanotechnology allows for the precise delivery of drugs directly to tumor sites, maximizing treatment effectiveness and minimizing side effects on healthy tissues. Nanoparticles can penetrate the microstructure of blood vessels to directly attack cancer cells, significantly reducing the adverse effects of chemotherapy or radiation therapy.

The convergence of these cutting-edge technologies is opening new doors to health recovery, advancing precision medicine and personalized therapies to unprecedented levels. With ongoing technological breakthroughs, the path to curing cancer is becoming increasingly clear.

Cutting-Edge Technologies In Cancer Diagnosis And Therapy: Innovative Breakthroughs Reshaping The Future Of Medicine

Next, we focus on several groundbreaking advancements that are bringing new hope to the field of cancer. The following notable examples and forward-looking recovery options are reshaping the future of cancer management:

Early Cancer Detection with Novelna Technology

In January 2024, U.S. researchers developed a diagnostic technology called Novelna, capable of detecting 18 types of early-stage cancers by analyzing blood proteins. In a screening of 440 cancer patients, the detection rates were 93% for male patients and 84% for female patients. Although still in its early stages, this technology lays the foundation for multi-cancer early detection in the future.

Advancements in AI: AlphaFold 3

In May 2024, Nature published the latest research on AlphaFold 3, an AI model developed by Google DeepMind. AlphaFold 3 can accurately predict protein structures and their interactions, marking a significant breakthrough in life sciences. This innovation is expected to revolutionize the diagnosis and treatment of diseases like cancer, further advancing AI's role in healthcare.

High-Precision Micronano Robots for Cancer Therapy

In July 2024, Harbin Institute of Technology unveiled a high-precision motile micronano robot based on neutrophils. These robots can navigate tiny blood vessels to deliver drugs precisely to cancer cells, significantly improving treatment accuracy while minimizing damage to healthy tissues. The research team has made substantial progress in using micronano robots for targeted cancer therapy.

Compared to the DNA nanorobots developed by the National Center for Nanoscience and Technology of the Chinese Academy of Sciences, Harbin's micronano robots have unique designs and working mechanisms. The DNA nanorobots employ self-assembling DNA structures that target tumor vasculature, delivering thrombin to induce vascular embolism and effectively suppress tumor growth. In contrast, Harbin's micronano robots utilize the natural chemotaxis and blood-brain barrier traversal capabilities of neutrophils combined with magnetic materials to enable precise treatment of brain tumors.

These two types of nanorobots, while differing in design concepts, working mechanisms, and application areas, reflect China's leading-edge exploration of cancer treatment with nanotechnology. They provide innovative approaches and possibilities for future precision cancer therapies.

AI Models for Tumor Diagnosis

Also in July 2024, Dr. Li Xiangchun from Tianjin Medical University published a study in Nature introducing an advanced AI model capable of identifying the primary site and characteristics of tumors with 98.9% accuracy. This technology significantly enhances the precision of cancer diagnosis and treatment, reducing the need for unnecessary surgeries.

AI-Powered Cancer Diagnosis: Groundbreaking Advancements of the CHIEF Model

On September 4, 2024, the Financial Times published an article detailing a groundbreaking AI model called CHIEF (Clinical Histopathology Imaging Evaluation Foundation), developed by a research team led by Kun-Hsing Yu, Assistant Professor at Harvard Medical School. This model analyzes digitized tumor tissue slides, enabling the precise identification of various cancer types, assessment of treatment efficacy, and prediction of patient survival rates.

Trained on large-scale datasets, the CHIEF model is capable of recognizing 19 different types of cancer, achieving an overall detection accuracy of nearly 94%. For certain cancers, including esophageal, gastric, colorectal, and prostate cancer, its accuracy reaches an impressive 96%. This highly efficient and precise analytical method provides strong support for clinical diagnosis and personalized treatment, demonstrating the immense potential of artificial intelligence in the medical field.

Ultra-High Dose Rate Electron Beam Therapy System by e-Flash

On November 7, 2024, Zhongjiu Flash Medical Technology Co., Ltd., a subsidiary of Changhong Group, unveiled its independently developed e-Flash Ultra-High Dose Rate Electron Beam Therapy System. This system is specifically designed for superficial tumors such as skin cancer and post-surgical residual lesions. Utilizing ultra-high dose rate electron beams, the device offers significant advantages, including drastically shortened treatment times and markedly reduced side effects. With an adjustable penetration depth ranging from 1 to 4 cm, the energy is precisely focused on the affected area, effectively sparing healthy tissues.

The e-Flash system compresses single treatment sessions to milliseconds, reducing the weeks-long traditional radiotherapy regimen to just a few sessions, each lasting under one second. This innovation represents a breakthrough in China's development and application of FLASH radiotherapy technology, offering new hope to cancer-affected individuals.

AI Model for Brain Tumor Detection by AITHYRA

On November 14, 2024, Austria's Die Presse reported that an AI model developed by the Vienna Institute of Biomedical Artificial Intelligence (AITHYRA) can detect brain tumors often overlooked during surgeries within ten seconds. This AI model allows surgical teams to identify tumors in seconds, enabling more precise excision, improving surgical success rates, and reducing the likelihood of recurrence. By leveraging advanced imaging technology and machine learning, the model enhances both the speed and accuracy of tumor detection. This innovation significantly improves surgical outcomes for brain tumors and positively impacts the prognosis of affected individuals.

Groundbreaking Advances in Plasma-Based Cancer Therapy Mechanisms

On November 15, 2024, the Hefei Institutes of Physical Science at the Chinese Academy of Sciences announced a significant breakthrough in the study of plasma-based cancer therapy mechanisms. The research demonstrated that low-dose atmospheric cold plasma (CAP) can effectively inhibit the growth of cancer cells. Further investigation revealed that the mechanism involves disrupting the structure and function of mitochondria within cancer cells, thereby inducing mitotic catastrophe and ultimately suppressing tumor growth. This discovery opens new possibilities for precision cancer therapy.

The study was funded by a key project of the National Natural Science Foundation of China, and the findings have been formally published in the internationally renowned journal Advanced Science. As an emerging therapeutic approach, cold plasma technology has shown a unique inhibitory effect on cancer cells, offering transformative insights into the future of cancer treatment.

HIFU Knife® High-Intensity Focused Ultrasound Therapy

The HIFU Knife® is China's first large-scale medical device with entirely independent intellectual property. This non-invasive treatment technology uses high-intensity focused ultrasound to precisely destroy tumor cells while maximizing the preservation of surrounding healthy tissues. HIFU technology has been widely applied as an adjunctive treatment for various malignant tumors, including liver cancer, pancreatic cancer, and kidney cancer. It is especially suited for individuals unwilling to undergo traditional surgery, those ineligible for surgery, or those with low surgical tolerance.

Non-Invasive Gastrointestinal Cancer Detection via Plasma 5hmC Biomarker

A collaborative effort by the First Affiliated Hospital of Anhui Medical University, the First Affiliated Hospital of Bengbu Medical College, Anhui Public Health Clinical Center, and Tailai Biosciences showcased a non-invasive method for detecting gastrointestinal cancers using plasma free 5hmC as a biomarker. This breakthrough has been recognized by the European Society for Medical Oncology Asia Congress (ESMO Asia) and published in the journal Annals of Oncology.

These groundbreaking technologies are revolutionizing cancer treatment, bringing new hope to cancer-affected individuals. Advances in science are gradually dismantling the traditional notion of cancer as incurable. Personalized therapies and precision medicine are emerging as the mainstream trends in future cancer recovery and treatment. These innovations illuminate a path of hope for all battling cancer, making the ultimate defeat of cancer an increasingly achievable reality.

The Wisdom of East and West: Breakthroughs in Integrative Medicine

Traditional Chinese Medicine (TCM), rooted in a holistic worldview, emphasizes harmony among the body, mind, and environment, focusing on internal balance and regulation. In contrast, Western medicine relies on modern technology and targets cancer cells directly. At different stages of cancer treatment, Western medicine can quickly suppress or eliminate tumors, while TCM supports recovery by alleviating treatment side effects, helping individuals better cope with pain, restoring physical strength, and improving overall quality of life.

As growing research confirms the effectiveness of integrative medicine in cancer recovery, this approach is gaining widespread recognition. Professor Li Ling of Peking University has noted that integrative medicine is likely to become a mainstream cancer treatment strategy in the future. By combining TCM's holistic regulation with the precision of Western medicine, a synergistic effect is achieved, offering comprehensive care for cancer patients. A core principle of TCM is enhancing the body's immune function to promote self-healing.

In August 2024, a study by Yale University in the United States demonstrated that traditional Chinese medicine (TCM) can effectively mitigate side effects from chemotherapy and radiotherapy, such as diarrhea, nausea, and fatigue, thereby improving patients' tolerance for treatment. This discovery underscores the immense potential of integrative medicine in cancer recovery. These groundbreaking findings position integrative therapies as a vital area of exploration in modern medicine, bringing renewed hope to cancer patients. By combining TCM and Western medicine, recovery outcomes are significantly improved, creating new possibilities in cancer treatment.

In recent decades, TCM has gained increasing scientific recognition. Numerous studies have tested the efficacy of TCM treatments like acupuncture and herbal remedies under controlled laboratory conditions, validating their clinical effectiveness. Many contemporary publications discuss the role of integrative medicine, particularly in treating chronic illnesses, cancer, and stress-related disorders. These findings highlight how the two medical systems complement each other to achieve better therapeutic outcomes.

The combination of the precision of modern medicine with the holistic regulation of TCM is gradually reshaping the way cancer is diagnosed and treated. Through this emerging recovery approach, many cancer patients not only achieve extended survival but also experience improved quality of life alongside medical intervention. This model introduces the concept of "living with cancer," shifting the focus from solely achieving a cure to emphasizing overall quality of life.

Integrative medicine offers not only more choices for cancer recovery but also new directions for the future of medicine. This combined treatment model leverages the scientific advancements of modern medicine while incorporating the personalized wisdom of TCM. The synergy between the two not only alleviates the suffering experienced during treatment but also boosts immune function, enhances quality of life, and ultimately empowers cancer patients to combat the disease more effectively, ensuring long-term health and well-being.

Comprehensive Therapies: A Holistic Support System for Healing

The success of cancer treatment lies not only in alleviating symptoms but also in addressing the underlying causes of the disease. This is particularly critical for managing advanced-stage cancers, where selecting the right intervention and timing is essential. Integrative therapies not only extend survival but also significantly enhance quality of life and recovery potential.

Through my journey battling cancer, I have gathered invaluable insights, with the following points standing out as especially

important:

1. Comprehensive Health Management

For many individuals confronting advanced cancer, physical pain, anxiety, and depression are often unavoidable. Comprehensive health support not only addresses physical symptoms but also provides emotional comfort and psychological well-being. Collaborative efforts by multidisciplinary medical teams bring together expertise from various fields, delivering holistic care and support throughout treatment.

2. Combining Medical and Complementary Therapies

Integrating conventional medical treatments with emerging technologies and the recovery strategies outlined in Chapter 5, along with lifestyle adjustments, reduces side effects and improves overall health. This dual approach enhances recovery outcomes and lays the foundation for long-term well-being. This combined strategy has provided a more positive recovery experience for myself and many others facing similar challenges, yielding remarkable progress.

3. Strengthening the Immune System

A primary objective of integrative recovery strategies is to fortify the immune system and elevate overall health. A robust immune system not only combats cancer cells more effectively but also enhances the efficacy of conventional recovery methods. By promoting the body's natural healing abilities, integrative therapies provide cancer-affected individuals with stronger defenses, making recovery a more attainable outcome.

4. Personalized Recovery Plans

The cornerstone of integrative recovery is personalization—tailoring strategies to meet individual needs, health conditions, and lifestyles. Personalized recovery plans address specific requirements, significantly improving outcomes and minimizing side effects. My own experience underscores the value of these tailored strategies, making the process more targeted and greatly increasing the likelihood of recovery.

5. Slowing Disease Progression

Certain integrative therapies have demonstrated remarkable efficacy in slowing disease progression. By optimizing cellular environments, reducing inflammation, and enhancing bodily functions, these approaches not only extend life but also improve overall health. I have personally experienced and witnessed the long-term benefits of these therapies, which have successfully arrested disease progression while significantly improving my physical condition and quality of life. Over the years, I have maintained a healthy lifestyle, moving forward steadily with normalcy in my daily life.

6. Emphasizing Mental Health

Integrative recovery strategies place significant importance on mental health. As discussed in Chapter 6, psychological recovery and inner strength are indispensable in this process. Psychological support helped me regain control over my health, enriching my overall life experience. Therapies combining physical treatment and psychological care ensure a positive mindset and steadfast determination when facing cancer, enhancing the immune response and overall resilience.

in summary, the organic combination of these elements creates a robust support system for individuals affected by cancer. This holistic health strategy equips people to better manage the challenges of cancer, significantly improving their quality of life while extending survival. Furthermore, it instills confidence and courage in the fight against cancer, greatly enhancing the chances of recovery and the potential for a cure.

Conclusion

This chapter not only highlights the complexity of cancer treatment but also underscores the pivotal role of a healthy lifestyle throughout the process. Furthermore, a positive mindset, mental well-being, and keen awareness of the body's signals are essential inner strengths in the battle against illness.

Recovery from disease relies not only on doctors and advanced medical technologies but also on an individual's steadfast commitment, full cooperation, and unwavering perseverance. Modern medicine offers us a wide range of strategies, but these can only achieve their full potential when actively embraced and pursued by the individual.

With hope and resilience, facing every challenge head-on, the advancements of science and the strength of the human spirit will ultimately help us conquer cancer. This chapter aims to instill confidence and convey the belief that the hope of recovery belongs to everyone—rebirth is not an unattainable goal. Though the path ahead may be fraught with challenges, it is equally filled with hope. Together, let us strive for a brighter, healthier future!

CHUNMEI YAO

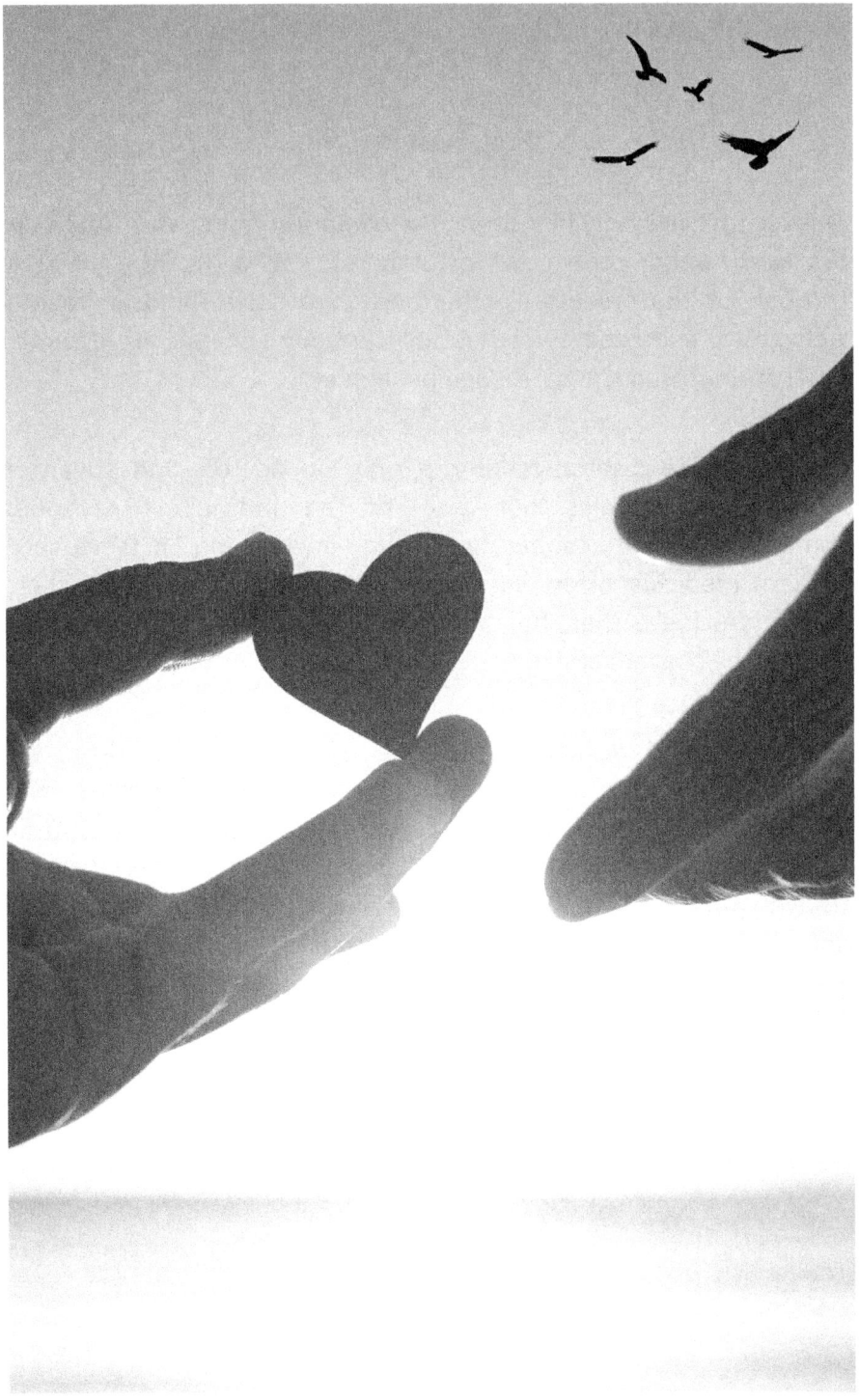

CHAPTER 10: THE GIFT OF HOPE AND WISDOM – REFLECTIONS AND SHARED INSIGHTS

In the darkest moments of life, stories of courage and healing remind us never to give up. These narratives ignite a spark of renewal, a radiant flame that fuels our determination to keep moving forward. Hope is not merely an emotion; it is a powerful driving force. When all other supports crumble, hope compels us to persevere.

For those battling life-threatening illnesses, holding on to hope can often mean the difference between surrender and resilience. I have personally experienced this: even when the path ahead is clouded with uncertainty, giving up must never be an option. Hope grants us the courage to confront daily challenges, inspires us to seize every opportunity in adversity, and encourages us to keep striving. It reminds us that healing is not impossible, even when the odds seem minuscule. This inner strength propels us to search for new avenues to survive, to trust in our capabilities, and to persist unwaveringly.

Our success stories are not merely personal triumphs; they stand as profound evidence of the possibility of recovery. Despite initial diagnoses that offered little hope, we chose to persevere. Through a combination of conventional medicine and natural therapies, we ultimately found a path to restored health.

Countless individuals around the world, facing seemingly hopeless circumstances, have triumphed over illness through unyielding faith and resilience. Such stories are far from rare; they not only inspire others but also highlight the complexity and richness of life, often surpassing our imagination. Healing sometimes emerges in unexpected ways—through breakthroughs in treatment, the support of faith and spirituality, or the selfless love of family and friends.

The journey to recovery teaches us that fostering belief is vital—not only for ourselves but also for those around us. Every reader of these stories should understand that even in the most challenging times, there is always a foundation of belief that sustains us. No matter how dire the circumstances, there is always a reason to press forward.

By sharing our experiences, we hope to help others discover their inner strength and believe in the possibility of recovery. Each of us has the power to spread positivity—whether through words of care, physical presence, practical assistance, or sharing our own stories. If you or someone close to you feels overwhelmed by a difficult diagnosis, remember: hope is ever-present. The strength of the spirit, the support of belief, and the resilience of personal will are often more powerful than we can imagine.

Every day is an opportunity to reignite hope; every battle brings us closer to victory. Do not hesitate to seek support—whether from family, friends, medical professionals, or alternative therapies. The journey to recovery, while challenging and uncertain, is also one of emotional growth, self-discovery, and personal fulfillment. Even when prognoses appear grim, miracles can still occur—such extraordinary turns of events can belong to anyone.

Thus, maintaining faith in recovery is crucial to physical healing.

This faith not only bolsters emotional and psychological resilience but also fosters a positive mindset, which can profoundly influence the effectiveness of treatment. Faith and hope help alleviate stress, bring inner peace and trust, and support the body's healing process on multiple levels. Believe in yourself, believe in the possibility of recovery—this is not only a celebration of life but also an anticipation of miracles.

A Guide for Supporting Those Affected by Cancer

Facing a cancer diagnosis, whether as a patient or a family member, emotional support and practical assistance are essential components of the recovery process. Understanding the illness and preparing mentally is the first step in the fight against cancer. In the most challenging moments, do not be intimidated by the life expectancy predicted by doctors. What matters most at this time is to regain composure, let go of psychological burdens, and focus on making every effort, avoiding the interference of fear and negative emotions, which can impair judgment, courage, and wisdom, as well as weaken decisiveness, confidence, and the motivation to persist.

No matter the stage of your physical condition, hope remains the driving force that propels you forward. By understanding the causes, symptoms, and coping strategies for cancer under the guidance of a professional doctor, there are always informed approaches to improve the chances of recovery. Taking time to research disease-related information, including coping methods and the latest scientific developments, can help build confidence, actively engage in the recovery process, and maintain an open mind to explore various possibilities. Since everyone's physical condition and response differ, finding the most suitable recovery path is crucial —whether through conventional medicine, alternative therapies, or other options that align with individual circumstances. Throughout this journey, closely monitor physical responses, record symptoms, and promptly adjust recovery and support plans in collaboration with medical professionals to achieve optimal results.

Improving your living environment and adjusting dietary habits are vital in balancing the immune system and helping the body enter a state more conducive to recovery. Every healthy choice is a significant step toward healing. This process can be long and fraught with challenges, and progress may not be immediate. However, perseverance, patience, and unwavering belief in the body's powerful ability to heal are critical.

Emotional support is equally indispensable. Ensure that you have people around who can provide emotional, practical, and spiritual support—be they family, friends, support groups, or professional advisors. The journey of fighting cancer need not be a solitary one; a strong support network can help you navigate the toughest moments. Open communication with family and friends about your feelings, fears, and needs can reduce misunderstandings and enable them to offer more effective support. Whether assisting with daily tasks or simply listening to you, their support becomes a vital pillar on your path to recovery.

Combining a belief in healing with a determination to seize every opportunity often leads to extraordinary outcomes. Anxiety and worry cannot change reality, but a positive mindset and joyful emotions can produce different results. Studies show that at least 85% of what we worry about never actually happens. Therefore, learning to live in the present and focusing on each moment can help us better and more efficiently navigate each day. Many troubles often stem from how we think and interpret situations.

During this time, steadfast belief and a positive attitude are essential. Cancer and its treatments exert immense emotional and physical stress. Employing effective stress management methods can help calm the mind. Finding what works best for you—whether it's exercise or other stress-reducing activities—is key. Whatever helps you most is the best choice.

Scientific studies have shown that maintaining a positive mindset stimulates the body to release endorphins, which help balance the immune system, promote recovery, and serve as a potent tool in fighting cancer. While fear and negative emotions are inevitable, choosing to respond positively can help you find inner strength during the toughest times. "Good emotions are the best 'anti-cancer medicine' and a form of 'positive energy.'" Many people discover that positive visualization and affirming statements can enhance mental strength and focus attention on the recovery process. Additionally, ensuring sufficient sleep and rest gives the body ample opportunities to recover—an integral part of the healing journey.

For family members and caregivers, patience and attentive listening are crucial. Your presence and care are the greatest support for those affected by cancer during their most difficult times. Loneliness, helplessness, and despair are their greatest enemies, while your love and support will help them overcome these challenges. At the same time, caregivers must not neglect their own physical and mental well-being, ensuring a healthy lifestyle for themselves and their loved ones.

By learning relevant knowledge, staying strong, and providing support for your loved ones, you can ease their burden and help them focus more on their recovery. Assisting with daily tasks can free up their time and energy for treatment. Engaging in meaningful activities together can divert attention, create cherished memories, reduce pain, and strengthen your bond.

Like many others, we have faced similar difficulties and ultimately achieved victory. We hope that this content inspires those currently facing similar challenges to move forward with courage, believing that they, too, can succeed. No matter the difficulties, each day is a new beginning, and every effort is a step closer to recovery. Trust in the power of miracles, believe in yourself, and embrace a brighter future.

The Importance of Daily Maintenance, Prevention, and Early Screening

A healthy lifestyle is one of the key factors in promoting physical recovery. Scientific studies have shown that good habits not only help prevent diseases but also significantly enhance overall health. However, many people neglect maintaining their health until a sudden illness reminds them of its importance. Some rely heavily on medication to sustain their well-being, but without improving lifestyle habits, even medical treatments may have limited efficacy.

For individuals with chronic illnesses, adhering to treatment plans while maintaining regular routines and a balanced diet can significantly improve their condition. Hospitals play a vital role in controlling the progression of diseases, but the key to recovery lies in an individual's sustained effort, commitment, and active cooperation. This is particularly true for those affected by cancer, as a healthy lifestyle can slow disease progression and provide robust support for treatment.

Although nutrition is not a substitute for medication, it plays an irreplaceable role in maintaining immune balance, promoting cell repair, and supporting overall recovery. While medical treatments are essential, nutritional support and healthy habits often enhance treatment outcomes and help prevent chronic disease or cancer recurrence. Thus, alongside medical intervention, personal lifestyle choices are indispensable elements in the recovery process.

Moreover, the human body possesses an extraordinary self-healing capability, which relies on the coordinated operation of multiple systems. With the support of the immune system, the body can identify and eliminate pathogens, repair damaged tissues, and maintain a healthy balance. Immunity and self-repair capacity are crucial in the recovery process, complementing medical treatments and laying the foundation for overcoming illness. The body's cellular renewal mechanisms also play a key role. Tissues such as skin, bones, and the liver have strong self-repair capabilities. When minor damage occurs, cells divide and regenerate to fill damaged areas and restore tissue function.

Scientific research indicates that the human body is composed of approximately 37 trillion cells, which maintain normal functions through continuous processes of apoptosis and regeneration. Every second, millions of cells die, while new ones are generated to replace aging or damaged ones. However, different types of cells have varying life cycles, and not all renew at the same rate. For example, red blood cells have a lifespan of about 3 to 4 months, skin cells renew every 2 to 4 weeks, and stomach lining and intestinal epithelial cells regenerate every 3 to 5 days.

In contrast, bone cells and some muscle cells renew more slowly. Most neurons in the brain cease renewal or regeneration after adulthood, though research suggests limited regeneration occurs in specific regions, such as the hippocampus. However, overall, brain cells have relatively limited recovery ability once damaged. Consequently, not all cells renew as frequently as those in the blood, skin, or digestive system.

After understanding the mechanisms of cellular renewal and their critical role in disease prevention, it becomes evident that maintaining good lifestyle habits is essential. These habits not only support normal cellular metabolism but also significantly enhance the body's self-repair capabilities. The health and renewal efficiency of cells largely depend on adequate nutritional supply, and a proactive lifestyle helps maintain the body in optimal condition, thereby promoting regular cellular renewal and functional recovery.

This aligns with the traditional Chinese medicine (TCM) principles of holistic health and the emphasis on prevention, encapsulated in the saying, "Food is better than medicine, and rest is better than food." It reflects the TCM philosophy of harmony between humans and nature, asserting that good lifestyle habits are the foundation of health. Modern scientific research supports this view: nutrition provides essential elements for cellular repair and regeneration, while adequate sleep and regular routines are crucial for the body's self-healing processes. Additionally, the nervous and endocrine systems play key regulatory roles in self-repair, influencing blood circulation, inflammatory responses, and cellular regeneration to help the body gradually recover.

For cancer, the stage at diagnosis significantly impacts survival rates. Early detection and the prompt formulation of suitable treatment strategies are key to successful outcomes. In the early stages, cancerous changes are often localized, without significant spread to other tissues or organs. This reduces the severity of harm and simplifies treatment, ultimately preserving the individual's quality of life. Prevention is better than cure; taking proactive measures in the early stages not only increases survival rates but also reduces treatment complexity. Maintaining a healthy lifestyle and undergoing regular checkups tailored to personal circumstances are effective ways to lower cancer risk. Preventive care should begin before the onset of illness, as it is more effective than attempting remedies after the disease has progressed. Early diagnosis, personalized treatment plans, and lifestyle management are critical to improving recovery rates.

Many people panic when they become ill, seeking medical intervention for minor discomfort. However, over-reliance on frequent checkups or screenings can lead to unnecessary issues, such as overdiagnosis, overtreatment, increased psychological stress, misdiagnoses, financial burdens, and disruptions to the body's natural balance. The human body is constantly changing, and mild discomforts often resolve on their own within days. Thus, instead of excessively relying on frequent checkup results, focus on overall bodily awareness. Every individual's health condition is unique, and standard metrics may not apply universally across all ages. For major disease diagnoses, seeking multiple opinions is crucial to ensuring accuracy and avoiding the psychological and financial strain of misdiagnoses.

As one of the success stories in this book, I can share my own experience. My cancer diagnosis in 2013 marked one of the darkest moments of my life, but fortunately, I recovered in 2016. However, just as I thought life was returning to normal, I encountered a terrifying misdiagnosis. The doctor's report sent me spiraling back to the emotional turmoil of 2013. Yet, having already battled cancer once, I responded calmly and rationally. I immediately sought further evaluations from three other specialists, which eventually confirmed that it was a false alarm. Since then, I have reduced my reliance on hospitals, placing greater trust in my body's signals. This decision proved wise, as I have enjoyed good health ever since and have not needed to visit a hospital again.

My experience illustrates that we should not let a single diagnosis dictate our emotions or decisions. Instead, we must learn to listen to our bodies and maintain confidence in our health while working collaboratively with doctors. By paying attention to bodily signals and responses, we can make wiser decisions when facing health challenges. With lifestyle improvements, the body naturally adjusts, and most minor discomforts represent normal physiological fluctuations that often resolve within days. However, for persistent or worsening symptoms, seeking timely medical help remains essential.

The impact of misdiagnoses on those affected by cancer is profound. Misdiagnoses can cause intense anxiety and confusion, potentially deteriorating mental health. Some individuals experience severe psychological stress, which may escalate into depression or other emotional disorders. In extreme cases, misdiagnoses can lead to hopelessness, resulting in tragic outcomes. Furthermore, misdiagnoses can erode trust in the medical system, making individuals skeptical of future diagnoses and treatments.

From a physical health perspective, misdiagnoses may lead to unnecessary medical interventions, such as surgeries or chemotherapy, resulting in severe side effects and delayed recovery. They can also impose significant financial burdens, affecting the quality of life for both individuals and their families. Thus, when faced with major illnesses, it is crucial to balance trust in doctors with cautious deliberation, seeking second or third opinions as needed. This approach not only helps maintain composure during critical moments but also fosters confidence in treatment decisions.

In daily life, the body often sends warning signals, but these signs are frequently overlooked. Regular self-examinations and attentiveness to physical changes are essential measures for disease prevention.

Cancer symptoms vary depending on the type and stage of the disease. Common warning signs include unexplained lumps or nodules, significant weight loss, physical weakness, persistent fatigue, chronic cough, prolonged pain, breathing difficulties, abnormal skin changes, digestive issues, bloating, difficulty swallowing, night sweats, lethargy, changes in bowel habits, or unexplained bleeding. If any of these symptoms occur, early screening is crucial to ensure timely detection and appropriate treatment interventions.

Prevention and early detection are critical in cancer recovery. While late-stage cancer can sometimes be cured, taking preventive measures early is far more effective in halting or slowing the progression of chronic diseases, significantly increasing the chances of successful treatment. Self-awareness, a balanced diet, moderate exercise, and avoiding harmful habits are all effective strategies for disease prevention.

Insights on Scientific Health Management from an International Medical Perspective

To better illustrate the importance of prevention in disease avoidance and control, we have referenced research and recommendations from medical experts, professors, and national health institutions in both China and the United States. These experts unanimously emphasize the pivotal role of daily health management and the cultivation of healthy lifestyle habits in disease prevention and cancer control. Their studies demonstrate that adopting scientifically grounded health practices can effectively reduce the risk of illness. Specifically, in the context of cancer prevention, their invaluable expertise further validates the significant impact of health management in substantially lowering the incidence of disease.

Authoritative Interpretations From Leading International Medical Institutions On This Topic

Harvard T.H. Chan School of Public Health

Harvard research has repeatedly highlighted the profound impact of a healthy lifestyle in reducing the risk of chronic diseases. Increasing daily physical activity and limiting the consumption of red meat and processed foods can effectively lower the incidence of cancers such as colorectal and breast cancer. Moreover, health management contributes to delaying the onset of various age-related diseases.

Centers for Disease Control and Prevention (CDC)

The CDC consistently emphasizes lifestyle interventions, such as smoking cessation, weight control, and increased physical activity, which have been proven to significantly reduce the prevalence of chronic illnesses, particularly cancer, cardiovascular diseases, and diabetes. By quitting smoking, limiting alcohol consumption, maintaining a healthy weight, and ensuring balanced nutrition, the risks of these related diseases can be substantially minimized.

Cancer Hospital, Chinese Academy of Medical Sciences

Oncology experts at this institution agree that adopting a healthy lifestyle is a vital approach to reducing cancer risk. While early screening and intervention remain critical, long-term health management—such as engaging in regular physical activity, managing psychological well-being, and maintaining dietary control—also plays a significant role in preventing cancer and mitigating its recurrence.

National Health Commission of China

This institution has long advocated for the prevention of chronic diseases through lifestyle improvements, aligning with China's public health policy objectives. Measures such as a balanced diet, moderate exercise, good sleep habits, and regular health checkups have proven effective in reducing the prevalence of chronic conditions, particularly major illnesses like cardiovascular diseases and cancer.

World Health Organization (WHO)

The WHO advocates for the global promotion of healthy lifestyles, underscoring the importance of prevention. By raising public awareness about health management—especially in the realms of cancer, diabetes, and hypertension—health education and daily preventive measures are recognized as some of the most cost-effective public health strategies worldwide.

Unique Perspectives From Experts And Professors On This Topic

Dr. Goobie, Neurosurgeon, USA

After resigning from a high-paying position in 2023, this 10-year veteran neurosurgeon shared his reflections on modern medicine via a short video in July 2024. He noted that while medical technology has achieved remarkable advancements in diagnosis and treatment, the focus on symptom management often neglects prevention and personal health management. He emphasized that many health issues can be effectively mitigated through early intervention and healthy lifestyles, reducing the need for medical interventions. This perspective does not diminish the importance of modern medicine but rather highlights the complementary roles of prevention, personal health management, and medical technology. By adopting proactive lifestyle changes, the risks of many chronic diseases can be significantly reduced, enhancing the effectiveness of medical treatments. His remarks sparked widespread discussion, encouraging individuals to balance reliance on medical advancements with daily health management and preventive measures.

Dr. Goobie further explained that many individuals endure prolonged back pain, neck pain, and neuropathy. While surgeries may provide temporary relief, they often fail to address the root causes. True recovery, he argued, requires a combination of dietary adjustments, improved sleep quality, mental relaxation, enhanced social interaction, appropriate exercise, and stretching. He particularly emphasized that the body's self-healing capabilities are the most effective means of recovery. As the body regains balance, other health issues, such as digestive function, gastrointestinal health, skin condition, and hair vitality, also tend to improve. This reflection has prompted many to reconsider the interplay between personal health responsibility and modern medical technology.

Dr. Yin Ye, CEO of BGI (Beijing Genomics Institute)

The progression from inflammation to tumors can take over a decade, with cancer often rooted in chronic inflammation. Therefore, anti-inflammatory measures and preventive medical testing are particularly crucial. Cancer does not arise suddenly; it is simply discovered suddenly. Early detection of tumors can prevent the suffering and complexity of late-stage cancer treatments.

Professor Li Ling, Peking University

"Health ultimately depends on oneself, while medical treatment is often supplementary." This simple yet profound statement underscores the importance of proactive health management, urging individuals to avoid excessive reliance on medical intervention and instead take responsibility for maintaining their own health.

Professor Shi Hanping, Director of Oncology, Capital Medical University

Nutritional therapy is the ultimate solution for managing all chronic diseases. Healthy eating is as crucial as radiation therapy, chemotherapy, and surgery. It is not merely a foundational method of recovery but also a vital component in addressing all illnesses. Nutritional support should be regarded as a cornerstone of treatment, capable of preventing and mitigating numerous unnecessary health risks.

Professor Tian Yantao, Chief Surgeon of Pancreatic and Gastric Surgery, Cancer Hospital, Chinese Academy of Medical Sciences

For those fighting cancer, proper nutritional intervention and maintaining a stable weight are not only essential for improving quality of life but also critical in overcoming cancer itself.

Professor Yu Kang, Clinical Nutrition Department, Peking Union Medical College Hospital

Nutrition plays not only a supportive role in disease treatment but also offers therapeutic and restorative effects, highlighting its irreplaceable value in clinical practice.

Professor Zeng Xianjiu, Renowned Chinese Surgeon

Many critically ill surgical patients do not succumb directly to their diseases but rather to malnutrition, which exacerbates their conditions. This highlights the paramount importance of adequate nutrition in critical care.

Academician Zhang Boli, President of Tianjin University of Traditional Chinese Medicine and Member of the Chinese Academy of Engineering

"Good habits are the foundation of health." He stressed that doctors cannot cure all diseases and that each individual should be their own best doctor. Health primarily relies on self-management and maintenance.

The information above, sourced from extensive research and public health advocacy by global authoritative institutions and experts, highlights the critical role of prevention and health management in reducing disease risks, controlling disease progression, and extending life expectancy. All these perspectives collectively emphasize the central role of nutrition, healthy lifestyles, and self-care in maintaining health and managing disease. Malnutrition can weaken the immune system, slow the healing process, and even lead to severe complications. Therefore, alongside conventional medical treatments, ensuring adequate nutrition for those affected by illness is crucial. These expert opinions further underscore the irreplaceable value of effective health management.

We cite these recommendations from professionals and institutions to help individuals integrate these insights into their daily lives, preventing and avoiding the onset of most diseases. However, if one day you are faced with the challenge of illness, the most important lesson is to face it courageously. Since certain realities cannot be changed, calmly accepting them and persevering is the key to overcoming adversity. This attitude often marks the beginning of a new life. Regardless of the stage of illness, maintaining a positive mindset is vital.

The Huangdi Neijing states: "Ninety percent of illnesses in the human body can heal themselves. When a person feels joy, the immune system becomes balanced, and energy pathways are unblocked." Thus, there is a saying: "A person's appearance changes every seven years, their complexion every seven days, and their spirit every seven minutes." This aligns with modern findings on the connection between mental health and the immune system. Contemporary science also confirms that positive emotions and mental states enhance immune function, enabling the body to better combat diseases.

The term "emotion" recurs throughout this book, clearly revealing its profound impact on physical and mental health. Chapter 6 particularly emphasizes the importance of emotions in physical recovery. During cancer treatment, excessive anxiety and uncertainty about the future can diminish focus, impair judgment, and even lead to poor decisions. When emotions are low, stress hormone levels in the body may rise, disrupting the normal functions of the nervous system and weakening the body's self-healing ability. Studies indicate that prolonged stress and negative emotions are closely associated with health issues such as obesity and cardiovascular disease.

In conclusion, preventing cancer and other chronic diseases requires a comprehensive approach that integrates biological, environmental, psychological, and social factors. Adopting holistic preventive measures not only reduces the risk of illness but also enhances recovery outcomes. Therefore, proper nutritional support, healthy lifestyle habits, and effective emotional management are not only essential for disease prevention but also accelerate the recovery process.

Boosting Energy and Rebuilding Health

When a person experiences prolonged fatigue, lethargy, dullness in the eyes, lack of vitality, and symptoms such as insomnia or forgetfulness, it often indicates a gradual decline in bodily functions. Studies show that low energy levels can lead to weakened immunity, making individuals more susceptible to infections and illnesses. Moreover, psychological well-being is closely tied to energy levels, with low energy often accompanied by symptoms of depression.

Individuals battling cancer frequently exhibit signs of energy depletion. This condition is driven by a combination of physiological and psychological factors, including the tumor's high energy demands, metabolic imbalances, chronic inflammation, malnutrition, and the overburdening of the immune system. In advanced stages of cancer, patients often experience pain, anemia, and abnormal energy metabolism. Cancer cells disrupt normal metabolic pathways in multiple ways, leading to inadequate nutrient absorption and exacerbating physical weakness.

All physiological activities in the human body rely on energy. Processes such as the beating of the heart, respiration, digestion, and cellular metabolism require a steady energy supply. Energy is the cornerstone of health, forming the foundation for the body's normal functions. Every cell depends on energy for metabolic activity, tissue repair, immune system support, cognitive function, and essential life processes. Adequate energy intake not only sustains daily activities but also plays a critical role in disease prevention, recovery, and overall health enhancement. Ensuring a sufficient and balanced energy supply is therefore vital to maintaining the body in optimal condition.

In traditional Chinese medicine (TCM), the key to boosting energy lies in the flow, balance, and nourishment of qi. Qi, regarded as the fundamental driving force of life, underpins the normal functioning of all physiological activities. By regulating qi and blood, balancing organ functions, and addressing harmony between environmental factors and emotional states, one can effectively enhance overall energy levels, improve physical resilience, and strengthen immunity. In this holistic framework, the unimpeded flow of qi and a balance between mind and body are inseparable. Only through internal and external harmony can the body achieve its optimal energy levels, fostering health maintenance and improvement.

The impact of energy replenishment on health extends beyond diet and physical functions to include emotional, psychological, and even spiritual dimensions. While healthy eating provides foundational energy, cognitive activities generate moderate energy, and higher levels of energy originate from elevated energy fields. When the body's energy field (e.g., biofield or qi field) is weakened, immune function declines, and emotional and psychological health are affected, increasing vulnerability to infections and illnesses.

Human energy is a tangible phenomenon. Higher energy levels correlate with greater inner strength, enabling individuals to fight cancer more resiliently and improve both their quality of life and life expectancy. Additionally, maintaining robust energy is a pathway to enhancing relationships, improving well-being, and adjusting one's overall trajectory in life. A strong and balanced energy field is therefore crucial for sustaining health and vitality.

Enhancing the body's energy requires a comprehensive approach, taking multiple factors into account. Below are some primary energy sources and their profound impacts:

Nutrition And Diet

As outlined in Chapter 5, nutritional support plays a vital role in improving overall health. Food serves as the primary source of vitality and energy, and a healthy diet forms the fundamental basis for maintaining the body's energy and vitality. Choosing fresh ingredients, high-quality foods, and maintaining a balanced diet can effectively enhance energy levels. Through healthy eating habits and a reasonable lifestyle, the body is better equipped to eliminate waste, thus improving its energy field.

From the perspective of dietary structure, apart from infancy, individuals across all age groups and health conditions require approximately 42 essential nutrients, categorized into six major groups. These nutrients are crucial for maintaining healthy physiological functions. However, specific nutritional needs vary depending on age and health status, and dietary structures should be tailored to the individual.

The essential nutrients typically include:

1. Proteins (composed of essential amino acids):

The building blocks for repairing and constructing body tissues.

2. Fats (essential fatty acids such as Omega-3 and Omega-6):

Critical for cell membrane structure, energy storage, and hormone production.

In October 2024, the International Journal of Cancer published a study indicating that the polyunsaturated fatty acids Omega-3 and Omega-6 may play a positive role in the prevention of various types of cancer.

3. Carbohydrates:

The primary energy source, particularly vital for brain and muscle function.

4. Vitamins:

Including water-soluble and fat-soluble vitamins, which are involved in metabolism, immune function, bone and skin health, blood clotting, and antioxidant activities. These ensure the body functions properly and is resistant to diseases.

5. Minerals:

Comprising macroelements and trace elements essential for energy metabolism and normal physiological functions. Foods rich in magnesium, iron, and B vitamins are especially important for energy metabolism and bone health.

6. Water:

While not traditionally classified as a nutrient, water is one of the key factors in maintaining health and energy levels. Chapter 5 also elaborates on the significance of hydration in the recovery process.

Additionally, it is crucial to minimize the consumption of high-sugar foods and processed products containing trans fats. These components can cause blood sugar fluctuations, leading to fatigue and reducing the body's energy levels.

By focusing on balanced nutrition and avoiding harmful dietary components, individuals can effectively sustain their energy, support physical resilience, and enhance overall health.

Sleep And Rest

Quality sleep is essential for restoring energy and serves as a fundamental pillar of health. The importance of sleep is an unavoidable topic in the fight against cancer, as emphasized throughout this book, particularly in Chapter 5, which discusses optimizing the sleep environment in detail. While rest is indispensable during illness, excessive rest may not necessarily aid recovery. Striking a balance between rest and activity is crucial for maintaining physical equilibrium.

Adults generally require approximately 7.5 hours of quality sleep each night to maintain mental clarity and alleviate fatigue effectively. However, individual sleep needs vary—some may require more sleep, while others may function well with less than 7.5 hours. Ideally, sleep should be scheduled between 10:00 PM and 6:00 AM, with deep, uninterrupted sleep between 11:00 PM and 5:00 AM being particularly critical. This window is when the body undergoes self-repair and regeneration, making it essential not to miss.

Good sleep hygiene also involves maintaining a consistent sleep schedule, creating a quiet and comfortable sleeping environment, and avoiding stimulating activities before bedtime. These include intense exercise, consuming caffeinated beverages, and using electronic devices, all of which can stimulate the nervous system and interfere with the ability to fall asleep. Reducing such disturbances allows the body to relax more quickly, promoting better sleep quality.

Tracking nightly sleep duration and assessing next-day alertness can help identify the optimal sleep routine. It is equally important to listen to the body's signals, engaging in a "dialogue" with it to understand its unique needs. Short naps or meditation can also serve as effective relaxation techniques, helping to relieve stress and restore energy. These practices are especially beneficial after periods of high-intensity work, providing the brain and body with necessary recovery time.

Maintaining a regular sleep schedule is vital for regulating the circadian rhythm, enabling the body to fall asleep at consistent times. This can enhance the quality of deep sleep, reduce unnecessary energy expenditure, and sustain stable energy levels. Furthermore, balancing work and life while managing time effectively ensures the preservation of energy. Overworking or enduring prolonged stress can deplete physical and mental resources, whereas appropriate leisure and relaxation promote energy restoration.

Physical Activity

Moderate and regular physical activity can boost energy levels by improving blood circulation, increasing oxygen supply, and stimulating the release of endorphins. Even short walks or light exercises can significantly enhance energy levels and improve mental health. Strength training and aerobic exercises, when combined, not only strengthen muscle function but also improve cardiovascular health, contributing to a notable increase in overall energy and endurance. However, it is essential to choose activities that best suit an individual's physical condition to achieve optimal results.

Emotional Strength And Social Support

In Chapter 8, we explored the critical role of mindset and mental well-being in coping with cancer. These factors are irreplaceable and cannot be overlooked. Psychological health profoundly influences energy levels, emotional stability, mental resilience, and overall vitality. Maintaining an optimistic outlook and practicing appropriate psychological adjustments are powerful forces in the recovery process.

A positive attitude is closely linked to energy levels. Chronic stress drains physical energy, leading to fatigue and burnout. While a positive mindset itself is not a direct source of energy, it indirectly enhances energy levels by reducing stress, improving mood, and promoting the release of endorphins and other "happiness hormones." Laughter, often referred to as "the best medicine," is an excellent way to boost energy. It not only alleviates tension but also improves mental health and helps restore physical balance.

Moreover, engaging in positive social interactions, such as connecting with friends and family, provides emotional and psychological energy. Such support enhances self-confidence, builds resilience, uplifts mood, and invigorates the spirit. Social activities stimulate cognitive functions, reduce feelings of loneliness, and lower stress levels, thereby improving overall energy states.

Building healthy relationships allows individuals to derive emotional satisfaction and psychological support from positive interactions, promoting balance and health. Positive emotions, a sound mental state, and supportive relationships contribute significantly to restoring and enhancing energy levels. Modern psychological research indicates that positive emotions, gratitude, a forgiving attitude, and strong social connections help reduce stress hormone levels and significantly improve mental energy and well-being.

Harnessing Natural Energy And Optimizing The Environment

Connecting with nature is one of the best ways to rediscover inner peace. Immersing yourself in the natural world, relaxing your body and mind, and taking deep breaths can help clear distractions, fostering balance and inner strength. For instance, exposure to morning sunlight and breathing in fresh air can effectively regulate the body's biological clock, significantly enhancing daytime alertness and vitality, thereby boosting overall energy levels.

Regular exposure to natural light promotes the normal secretion of melatonin at night, improving sleep quality. A healthy circadian rhythm is the foundation of restful sleep—a natural mechanism often overlooked. Spending time outdoors or taking brief breaks in nature during the day can significantly improve energy levels. Natural surroundings help restore baseline energy and promote balance between body and mind. According to an article in the internationally renowned Daily Science, just 20 minutes of daily exposure to nature can alleviate fatigue and anxiety while enhancing mental resilience.

No matter how advanced technology becomes, nature remains one of the purest, most miraculous, and most powerful sources of energy. Moderate activity in fresh air not only uplifts the mood but also replenishes the body with renewed vitality by absorbing nature's essence. Traditional Chinese medicine and health practices such as yoga view breathing exercises as a way to manage and enhance vital energy, emphasizing harmony between one's breath and the natural environment.

Sunlight, air, and vegetation in nature work together to regulate the body's energy field, restoring balance. Inhaling fresh oxygen nourishes cells while naturally generating energy. Thus, nature provides an unparalleled external source of replenishment, helping individuals return to a state of physical and mental harmony.

Gazing at blue skies and white clouds, or the stars and moon, evokes a sense of the universe's vastness and tranquility. This boundlessness seems to embrace all human emotions and desires, offering profound solace and gentle release. Such expansive scenes cleanse the soul, momentarily erasing worldly worries and instilling a rare sense of peace, as if stepping into a state of timeless serenity.

The Huangdi Neijing (Yellow Emperor's Inner Canon) notes that aligning oneself with the essence of nature—its sunlight and cosmic energy—helps restore bodily energy balance. Sunlight enhances yang energy, disperses dampness, and replenishes vitamin D, boosting overall vitality and immunity. In traditional Chinese medicine, this natural absorption of earth and celestial energies is called Heavenly Nourishment, a vital force bestowed by nature for maintaining health.

As for Earthly Nourishment, this is achieved through engaging with the tangible aspects of nature. Activities such as mountain climbing, admiring sea clouds from a summit, strolling through forests, or embracing ancient trees allow individuals to reconnect with the earth. Simple acts like touching leaves or appreciating flora can ground the mind, fostering a sense of presence and tranquility while restoring energy. When the weather permits, walking barefoot on soft soil or grass, or lying on a meadow basking in sunlight and breezes, helps the body harmonize with the earth's energy, promoting relaxation and yin-yang balance.

Standing by the sea, gazing at the endless blue, quietly admiring the sunset-painted sky, or walking barefoot along a soft sandy beach can feel like unburdening the soul and absorbing nature's nourishment. Listening to the rhythm of raindrops tapping the earth, feeling the gentle caress of the breeze, or taking firm steps beneath your feet—all these sensory experiences invite closer connections with nature, reawakening a deep-seated vitality. As traditional Chinese medicine suggests, living in harmony with seasonal changes and balancing yin and yang by integrating oneself with nature is key to holistic health. In reconnecting with the natural world, we can realign our energy fields and rediscover inner peace and harmony.

On the human nourishment side, choosing seasonal foods to absorb nature's essence, wearing attire that boosts confidence, maintaining a neat appearance to exude vitality, and surrounding oneself with uplifting, like-minded friends or spending time with positive individuals all contribute to replenishing and enhancing internal energy reserves. This lifestyle fosters gradual restoration of strength and inner power, aligning seamlessly with the upcoming discussion on enhancing mental energy through positive social interactions.

Additionally, reducing environmental disturbances is crucial. In both work and life, clutter and noise quietly drain energy and undermine focus. Tidying unused items and donating them to those in need not only keeps the surroundings orderly but also creates a clearer, more organized space. This process of decluttering lightens the psychological burden, enhances concentration, and promotes a more relaxed and energized state, leading to significant improvements in overall quality of life.

Spiritual Practice And Metaphysics: Bridging Inner Growth And Universal Harmony

Spiritual practice enhances inner energy, promoting psychological balance and emotional stability. These practices not only help alleviate stress but also strengthen the body's self-healing capabilities. For many, spiritual growth or rediscovering the meaning of life significantly amplifies vitality. This process brings peace and insight on a spiritual level, enriches emotional experiences, enhances psychological resilience, and ultimately boosts overall life force. Such practices have profound impacts on both mind and body, helping individuals better navigate the stresses and challenges of life.

The strength of one's energy field is influenced by the

integrated regulation of body, mind, and spirit. Beyond the physical benefits mentioned earlier, meditation, breathwork, and mindfulness practices are effective in harmonizing the overall energy field. Through these practices, individuals can not only connect with their inner strength but also enhance self-awareness and unlock potential, enabling them to maintain peace, faith, and resilience when faced with challenges. Meditation and breathwork, in particular, form the core elements and essential components of spiritual practice.

When discussing spirituality, metaphysics is an inevitable topic. Rooted deeply in Chinese traditional culture, metaphysics involves exploring the essence of the universe, life, and the principles that underlie them. In Chinese philosophy, particularly in Taoism and Confucianism, the relationship between humans, nature, and the universe is regarded as a key to maintaining health and harmony. One of the goals of spiritual practice is to achieve inner balance by fostering harmony with the universe. As the German philosopher Immanuel Kant once said, "Two things fill the mind with ever new and increasing admiration and awe, the more often and steadily we reflect upon them: the starry heavens above me and the moral law within me." This process reflects the pursuit of internal and external harmony.

The essence of this profound statement lies in the idea that while humans live within the vast physical universe, they must possess the ability for self-restraint and adhere to elevated ethical principles. The starry heavens and moral law, as eternal and uncontrollable existences, guide us to contemplate the meaning of life on moral and rational grounds, as well as the role we ought to play in the cosmos, thereby uncovering the true value of our existence. Kant's reflections on the "starry heavens" and "moral law" evoke a profound reverence for the self, the world, and higher ideals, mirroring the concept of "harmony between heaven and humanity" found in Chinese culture. Both transcend individual interests, pointing to higher principles that guide humanity in finding belonging and purpose within the universe and society.

Ancient Chinese thought posits that humans and the universe share an inherent harmony. The cosmos is seen as an ordered and sacred whole, and humanity is expected to align itself with the principles of the universe. Both Confucianism and Taoism emphasize this harmonious relationship. Taoism identifies the essence of the universe as the profound "Tao"—both the law governing natural operations and the code of conduct for humanity. Confucianism, on the other hand, advocates for achieving harmony between heaven and humanity through moral cultivation.

Thus, Kant's concepts of the "starry heavens" and "moral law" align remarkably well with the Chinese philosophical ideals of the "Way of Heaven" (Tian Dao) and the "Way of Humanity" (Ren Dao). This convergence reminds us that, whether in the East or the West, the reverence for and reflection upon both the universe and the self remains a shared spiritual pursuit of humankind.

While spiritual practice and metaphysics have different focuses and approaches in exploring the essence of life and the mysteries of the universe, they complement each other to some extent. This connection is also reflected in the discussion on sleep environments in Chapter Five of this book. Spiritual practice emphasizes personal inner experiences and self-awareness, aiming to achieve inner balance through mental regulation, thereby improving physical and mental health. In contrast, metaphysics explores spiritual phenomena, supernatural occurrences, and metaphysical principles through symbolic systems and philosophical inquiry.

For some, spiritual practice is not only a means to achieve better health but also a crucial pathway for personal growth and the development of inner strength. Metaphysics, on the other hand, offers a framework for understanding life, helping individuals calmly and rationally navigate major life changes by interpreting symbols and metaphors. The integration of spiritual practice and metaphysics provides dual support on both emotional and rational levels, enabling individuals to maintain inner peace and resilience when facing stress.

When examining the effects of spiritual practice and metaphysics on health, studies indicate that these approaches enhance mental energy and positively influence physical health, particularly in cellular health and aging mechanisms. As discussed in the previous section, the human body is in a constant state of metabolism, with cells aging, dying, and regenerating. Telomeres play a critical and decisive role in this process. These protective structures at the ends of chromosomes prevent damage during replication. However, telomeres shorten with each cell division. Once they reach a critical length, cells cease dividing and enter a state of senescence or apoptosis, a key mechanism in cellular aging and functional decline. Healthy diets and positive lifestyle choices can slow telomere shortening, supporting cellular health and delaying the aging process. Numerous scientific studies have confirmed that an active lifestyle helps maintain longer telomeres.

Additionally, spiritual practices have been found to slow telomere shortening, delay aging, and support cellular repair and recovery. A study published in Molecular Psychiatry revealed that long-term meditators exhibit longer telomeres, suggesting that meditation helps preserve telomere integrity and promote cellular health by reducing psychological stress and inflammation levels. Meditation, therefore, serves as a pathway to spiritual awakening and personal growth.

In general, healthy diets, regular exercise, stress management, sufficient sleep, and avoiding harmful habits contribute to delaying telomere shortening, promoting cellular health, and slowing aging.

Numerous studies have demonstrated that a proactive lifestyle helps maintain longer telomeres, supporting overall health.

In summary, spiritual practice and metaphysics provide valuable tools for many people to manage stress, offering methods to achieve inner balance and regulate emotions. They promote harmony between mind and body, serve as vital psychological support systems, and have a positive impact on health. These practices enable individuals to better navigate life's challenges, adopt healthier lifestyles, and indirectly or directly improve physical well-being. Furthermore, the positive effects of spiritual practices have been validated by multiple scientific studies, which show that long-term spiritual engagement fosters internal and external harmony, offering robust support and protection for physical and mental health. These practices encourage individuals to listen to their body's needs, focus on their well-being, and adjust their routines flexibly to suit their unique requirements.

Purification Of The Mind And Energy Enhancement

"Dāna" is a concept in Buddhism that transcends mere acts of charity, serving as a form of spiritual practice that elevates one's inner self in daily life. The practice of dāna purifies the mind, cultivates compassion, reduces attachment to material possessions, and fosters care for others, thereby achieving a higher level of personal growth. By generously offering resources, knowledge, time, or love within one's capacity, individuals not only assist others but also diminish greed, nurture compassion and wisdom, and accumulate merit. In Buddhism, dāna is regarded as a fundamental path to building good karma and achieving spiritual virtues.

While dāna bears some resemblance to the secular concept of "donation," the two are not entirely synonymous. On the motivational and spiritual levels, dāna emphasizes inner cultivation of compassion and is an integral part of Buddhist practice, whereas donation is more often a social act of goodwill.

In comparison, donations usually involve material or financial aid and may stem from altruism or a desire to help others, but they lack the spiritual and religious significance inherent in dāna. Moreover, donations might sometimes be accompanied by expectations, such as the hope to assist others or gain social recognition.

Dāna also enhances energy, not only on a physical level but also as a boost to mental and spiritual vitality. This increase in energy is reflected in several key aspects:

1. Reduction of Negative Emotional Drain

Dāna alleviates attachment and greed while preventing unnecessary emotional consumption. A selfless mindset fosters peace and relaxation, thereby accumulating positive energy.

2. Cultivation of a Positive Mindset

The act of giving benefits both the recipient and the giver, who experiences the joy and satisfaction of generosity. These positive emotions elevate psychological energy and overall happiness.

3. Strengthening Mental Resilience

Dāna nurtures compassion and empathy, enhancing mental resilience and tolerance. This inner strength enables individuals to face life's challenges with greater fortitude, reducing the energy drain caused by stress and anxiety.

4. Attracting Cycles of Positive Energy

The practice of dāna brings inner fulfillment and tranquility, fostering spiritual growth. It also tends to attract more positive energy and favorable connections, further raising overall energy levels.

5. Promoting Physical Health

By fostering a positive mental state, dāna helps reduce stress hormones and indirectly enhances physical vitality.

In summary, dāna not only elevates spiritual energy but also empowers individuals to better handle life's challenges, supporting holistic development of physical and mental health. For the average person, acts of giving and donation hold profound significance. They provide tangible support and warmth to others while allowing the giver to experience the joy of sharing and generosity.

Studies suggest that positive actions and emotions, such as helping others or expressing generosity, activate the body's "happiness hormones" like endorphins, serotonin, and oxytocin. These hormones not only bring emotional satisfaction but also boost energy levels, leaving individuals feeling invigorated. Such acts nourish the hearts of both giver and recipient, fostering a profound sense of fulfillment and happiness, which indirectly enhances vitality and overall well-being.

Prudent Use Of Medications

Medications play a critical role in treating certain illnesses. However, excessive reliance on them while neglecting lifestyle adjustments may hinder the enhancement of overall energy levels, as discussed in the previous section. Medications are often effective in alleviating symptoms and addressing specific causes of illness. Yet, achieving optimal health requires integrating medical treatment with a healthy lifestyle. Relying solely on medications may not fully improve energy and health; in some cases, it can negatively impact the body's natural functions, such as weakening immunity, reducing energy levels, and impairing self-healing abilities.

Reducing long-term dependence on medications while adopting a healthy lifestyle can enhance the body's natural defense mechanisms and energy reserves, leading to more comprehensive health and energy management. Therefore, a combined approach is key to improving overall health and optimizing energy levels. Any adjustments to medication use should be made under medical supervision to ensure safety and efficacy. Additionally, under professional guidance, natural remedies such as herbal supplements like Lingzhi (reishi mushroom) and ginseng can be considered to restore and enhance energy, though their use must be tailored to individual constitutions.

This section explores various methods to elevate physical energy, promote holistic health, improve quality of life, and experience a deeper sense of well-being. Life's essence is energy, and cultivating energy awareness while continuously enhancing energy levels is essential. Energy manifests through multiple dimensions, including diet, nature, psychological well-being, social connections, and spirituality, all of which play vital roles in maintaining health and facilitating recovery. By balancing these forms of energy, the body's self-healing capacity can be significantly strengthened, providing robust support for overall health and recovery. This multi-dimensional approach not only enhances vitality but also offers a powerful inner strength to face life's major challenges.

Maintaining and balancing these energies is crucial for holistic health improvement and disease resistance. It not only builds emotional and psychological resilience but also brings about positive physical and spiritual transformations. An individual's energy state is the result of complex interactions among various factors, making it particularly important to adopt an integrative approach to address and improve this state.

Letting Go For Energy Renewal

In addition to the energy sources mentioned earlier, an effective way to recharge is by fully relaxing the mind, clearing one's thoughts, and aligning with nature without clinging to things beyond one's control. This is particularly important when dealing with negative emotions or challenging people and situations. Maintaining a non-reactive stance helps conserve energy and preserve inner balance. Only when external disturbances completely subside, and inner tranquility is achieved, can one reach a vibrant and empowered state of being.

Moreover, through comprehensive adjustments to the body, mind, and spirit, one can promote the evolution of both conscious and subconscious awareness, potentially unlocking latent potential and enhancing the flow of life energy. When the body is filled with energy, physical health improves, joy arises from within, clarity of thought prevails, and relationships naturally become more harmonious. This state naturally attracts positivity, fostering good fortune and even altering the trajectory of one's destiny. Energy functions like a magnetic field: the stronger the energy, the healthier the body and mind become, while negative energy and illness gradually fade away. Many misfortunes in life stem from internal imbalance, but when the heart is filled with light and one's energy field is strong enough, even in the midst of darkness, the light of hope remains visible.

Embracing Tolerance And Wisdom

When an individual elevates their energy to a higher level, they begin to understand the principles underlying the workings of the world. They realize that there is no absolute right or wrong, good or bad in life. The differences in perspectives, attitudes, and choices arise from variations in individual viewpoints and frequencies, leading to discrepancies in understanding and judgment.

Therefore, learning to accept oneself, living authentically, and respecting others' ways of life while acknowledging their unique existence reflects profound tolerance and wisdom. This form of acceptance is not only a sign of respect for oneself and others but also a testament to a deep understanding of life's essence and harmonious coexistence.

Essential Principles for Enhancing Cancer Recovery

No matter the challenges faced by individuals affected by cancer, maintaining hope, seeking support, gaining knowledge, and staying surrounded by family and friends can bring about profound changes, enabling recovery and a return to health. To better encourage those battling illness and provide practical guidance, this section outlines several key principles for combating cancer. These core ideas are designed to empower individuals during difficult times, instilling strength and confidence as they navigate the journey toward recovery.

These principles encompass the core strengths for confronting cancer and are outlined as follows:

1. Cancer Is Not the End

A cancer diagnosis is not the end of life but rather an opportunity to reexamine its meaning. While the illness may test your resolve, it can also serve as a chance for renewal. The true motivation for recovery should stem from your inner strength. Remember, everything in life happens for a reason—it is either a gift or a lesson.

2. Acceptance of Reality

Acknowledging the current reality of illness helps reduce psychological stress, allowing focus on what can be controlled. Acceptance fosters a rational approach to managing the disease and enhances recovery prospects.

3. Will to Live and Self-Confidence

A cancer diagnosis often marks the beginning of an emotionally profound journey. The desire to live and a strong will to survive are at the heart of overcoming cancer. Trust in yourself and your body's capabilities can unleash immense inner energy, strengthening the immune system and enabling active participation in the recovery process.

4. Unwavering Belief

Belief plays a decisive role in critical moments. A steadfast belief sustains the will to survive, even in the most challenging times. While the support of doctors and others is invaluable, you are the primary driver of your own health. Believing in the possibility of miracles provides ongoing strength and keeps you resolute in pursuing recovery.

5. Emotional Management

Negative thoughts are a person's greatest adversary. Maintaining a positive mindset boosts inner strength. Fighting cancer requires not only modern medical treatments but also an optimistic attitude and life approach. In adversity, discover the strength to move forward, tap into inner potential, and build psychological resilience. This power will support you through every stage of the journey, bringing transformative results.

6. Inner Spirit and Faith

The inner spiritual strength or faith you hold can offer immense comfort and support. During the fight against illness, this strength shields you from succumbing to external difficulties.

7. Determination to Persevere

In the battle against cancer, enduring resilience and unwavering determination are crucial. Confronting setbacks and pain with a resolute spirit enables you to persevere and ultimately conquer the disease.

8. Support and Empathy

The emotional support of family and friends plays a pivotal role in recovery. Social support improves mood, reinforces the motivation to overcome illness, and provides a sense of love and encouragement.

9. Self-Care

A healthy lifestyle and self-management are critical in coping with cancer. By prioritizing self-care, you can improve your physical condition, enhance immune function, and better combat the disease.

10. The Power of Nature

Respect the healing potential of nature and trust in your body's innate ability to heal. Combining natural wisdom with modern medicine creates optimal conditions for recovery.

11. Miracles of Healing

Your journey is not unique—many others have overcome seemingly insurmountable challenges through persistence and courage. Their recovery is a testament to the miraculous self-healing power of the human body.

In summary, the most effective way to face cancer is to release psychological burdens, confront and accept reality, and adopt tailored strategies for healing. Once mentally prepared, taking proactive and deliberate action often yields better results. This principle is discussed in detail in Chapter Six. Prioritizing recovery should take precedence, with other concerns temporarily set aside. Another critical point is not to view yourself solely as a patient. Stay occupied with daily tasks, arrange meaningful activities, or complete goals you may have postponed before falling ill. This helps maintain inner peace and effectively reduces fear and anxiety, which in turn supports recovery.

The above principles represent essential inner strength, self-care strategies, and the immutable laws of nature when confronting illness. By adhering to these beliefs, you will demonstrate the resilience and courage needed to overcome cancer and embrace a brighter future.

When you succeed in defeating illness, you will, like many others, gain a fresh perspective on life and begin a new chapter, enriched by newfound strength and insight.

Conclusion

This chapter has explored multidimensional health strategies, demonstrating how psychological strength, physical energy balance, social support, spiritual resilience, and harmony with nature can collectively form a robust support system when facing significant health challenges like cancer. Health is not merely the outcome of medical treatment; it is a holistic approach to life and a practice of cultivating the mind and spirit.

Healing from cancer is not only about physical recovery but also about spiritual growth. By emphasizing the multifaceted role of energy—from physical to psychological and spiritual dimensions—this chapter highlights the indispensable contributions of each aspect to bodily recovery and overall well-being. Whether through connection with nature or social interactions, these sources of energy play a vital role in enhancing vitality and supporting the healing process.

The power of the mind and the balance of energy are essential tools in the fight against illness. Maintaining optimism, steadfastly battling disease, and seeking meaning in life can illuminate the path for every individual on their journey toward a healthier and more fulfilling future.

Happiness and inner peace stem from understanding oneself and one's destiny. It is essential to focus on what can be influenced and to improve life through proactive actions. At the same time, learning to accept what cannot be controlled is equally important. This ability not only fosters inner balance and tranquility but also allows for better concentration on achievable goals. It is a crucial step toward maturity and inner harmony. Often, what troubles us is not the situation itself but our perception of it. This mindset provides profound insight when facing difficulties, stress, and challenges, helping us approach life's storms with a better attitude. Ultimately, what determines your health is not solely doctors or medical treatments, but your actions and choices. Each daily decision and commitment to a healthy lifestyle lays the foundation for your recovery journey.

With this, the book has comprehensively discussed the experiences and strategies for overcoming cancer and other challenges through various balancing methods. For readers who wish to explore further, the book includes academic resources and references for additional study.

Finally, we conclude with a philosophical reflection:

"The potential for health in the body is limitless; the real challenge is convincing your mind."

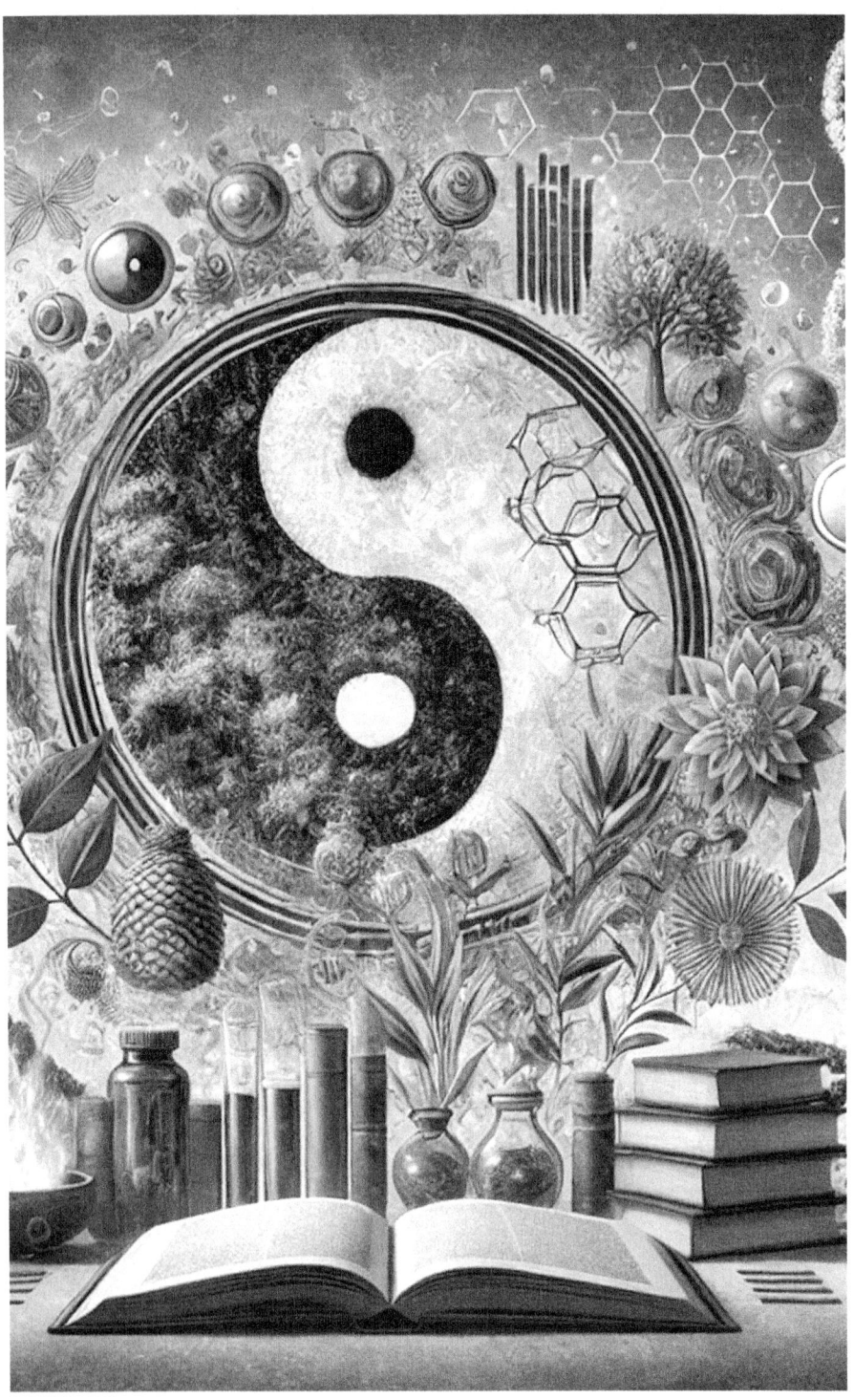

CHAPTER 11 : ACADEMIC RESOURCES AND REFERENCES – SCIENTIFIC KNOWLEDGE AND SUPPORT FOR HEALTH

This chapter compiles a wealth of significant studies, reference materials, links, and other relevant resources that have guided us throughout the journey of combating cancer. These resources are derived from authoritative academic research and medical practices, encompassing the causes of cancer, modern treatment methods, recent research developments, and future prospects. They have provided critical support in our fight against cancer.

We deeply understand the importance of these resources in the recovery process. By listing them here, we hope to help readers gain a deeper understanding of cancer-related knowledge, inspire others battling the disease, and offer new perspectives and solutions.

These resources not only reflect the progress of medicine and science but also embody the wisdom and resilience of humanity in the face of illness. Exploring these materials can empower you to make more informed decisions and strengthen your confidence in overcoming the disease.

The specific related information is as follows:

Key Reference Book

The China Study

Authors: T. Colin Campbell and Thomas M. Campbell II

The China Study is a large-scale, highly influential epidemiological study exploring the relationship between diet, lifestyle, and the incidence of various diseases. As one of the most extensive and detailed studies of its kind to date, it has garnered significant attention and sparked widespread discussion in the global nutrition community.

This study highlights the profound impact of diet on health, particularly concerning chronic diseases such as cancer, heart disease, and diabetes. The findings indicate that regions where plant-based diets are predominant have significantly lower rates of chronic diseases compared to regions where animal-based diets are more common.

Beyond dietary factors, The China Study also considers other lifestyle elements, such as smoking, physical activity, and environmental conditions, which similarly play crucial roles in health outcomes.

The study has had a far-reaching influence on public health discussions, providing robust scientific evidence for the benefits of plant-based diets. Frequently cited as a foundational text for advocating healthy eating, it has deepened understanding of the connection between diet and disease prevention. The China Study has made significant contributions to recognizing the role of nutrition in disease prevention and offers a solid scientific basis for those seeking to improve health through dietary changes.

Important Online Resource Links

Pubmed

A Vital Resource for Biomedical and Health Sciences Research

https://pubmed.ncbi.nlm.nih.gov/

PubMed is a comprehensive, free online database that provides access to a vast collection of scientific literature in the fields of biomedicine, life sciences, and health sciences. It serves as an essential tool for researchers, healthcare professionals, and academics worldwide, enabling them to access both recent and historical studies. The database includes millions of articles from various authoritative journals, covering topics such as medical research, life sciences, clinical trial reports, and systematic reviews. PubMed has become indispensable for professionals seeking to stay updated with global research advancements.

The content available on PubMed spans multiple disciplines, including medicine, pharmacology, nursing, public health, and molecular biology. While most publications are in English, the database also includes articles in other languages. PubMed provides abstracts for many studies and links to full-text articles, some of which are freely accessible. However, not all articles are available for free, requiring users to access them through institutional subscriptions or purchase.

Despite these limitations, PubMed remains an invaluable repository of knowledge, offering researchers worldwide access to cutting-edge scientific information. By facilitating the dissemination of knowledge, PubMed continues to drive progress in medicine and health sciences.

Phoenix Tears

A Resource for Exploring the Potential of Medicinal Cannabis

www.phoenixtears.ca

Phoenix Tears is a website founded by Rick Simpson, a renowned Canadian advocate for medicinal cannabis. He is widely recognized for promoting the potential of "cannabis oil," also known as Rick Simpson Oil (RSO), in cancer recovery. Rick Simpson claims to have cured his own skin cancer using homemade cannabis oil, a remarkable experience that has made him a steadfast proponent of the medical value of cannabis.

On the Phoenix Tears website, you can find detailed instructions for making and using Rick Simpson Oil, including recommended dosages and usage guidelines. The site also features numerous success stories, sharing positive outcomes from individuals who have used cannabis oil in their recovery journey.

It is important to note that, while many users have reported benefits from cannabis oil, its use should ideally be undertaken under medical supervision, with careful consideration of potential risks. Phoenix Tears serves as a valuable resource for understanding the supportive potential of cannabis oil, but caution and critical thinking are essential when considering this therapy.

Salvestrol Capsules

https://www.kingnature.ch/content/uploads/salvestroleneue_moeglichkeiten_der_krebsbehandlung.pdf

Article Link: Salvestrols - New Possibilities in Cancer Adjunct Therapy

This article, published in 2009 in the Journal of Orthomolecular Medicine & Nutrition (OM & Nutrition), is based on research conducted by Professor Dan Burke and Professor Gerry Potter. It explores the potential applications and findings of Salvestrols in cancer adjunct therapy.

Key Findings of Salvestrol Research

British scientists have discovered that Salvestrols can activate the CYP1B1 enzyme in cancer cells, leading to the selective death of these cells. This groundbreaking discovery offers new hope for cancer recovery.

The widespread use of modern agricultural techniques has significantly reduced the levels of Salvestrols in food. The use of pesticides, in particular, has suppressed the natural need for plants to produce these protective toxins, resulting in a decline in Salvestrol intake.

The critical role of nutrition is further highlighted, with studies suggesting that choosing organic foods and increasing Salvestrol intake may help reduce the risk of cancer and serve as an adjunct to existing cancer treatments.

Research also indicates that the CYP1B1 enzyme is overexpressed in almost all human cancers, making it a universal tumor marker. This finding underscores the significant potential of Salvestrols as a targeted therapeutic tool that exclusively acts on cancer cells.

Relevant Research and Practical Overview

Studies On Turmeric And Black Pepper

The Synergistic Effects of Curcumin and Piperine

Shoba, G., et al. (1998)

Published in: Planta Medica, 64(4), 353–356

This study demonstrated that the combination of curcumin (from turmeric) and piperine (from black pepper) significantly enhances the bioavailability of curcumin, with an increase of up to 2000%. This enhancement prolongs the retention of curcumin in the body, thereby amplifying its therapeutic effects. The research delves into the biochemical synergy between curcumin and piperine, providing a scientific basis for their combined use to maximize health benefits.

Curcumin's Inhibition of Cytochrome P450 and Potential Drug Interactions

Plummer, S.M., et al. (1999)

Published in: Biochemical Pharmacology, 58(4), 819–825

This study found that curcumin inhibits certain types of the cytochrome P450 enzyme system, potentially affecting the metabolism of other drugs. This discovery is particularly relevant for individuals taking multiple medications, as curcumin may enhance or prolong the effects of these drugs. Therefore, caution is advised when combining curcumin with other medications to avoid potential drug interaction risks.

Key Insights

These two studies highlight the synergistic effects of curcumin and piperine, which significantly improve the supportive benefits of curcumin. Additionally, they reveal the potential risk of curcumin affecting drug metabolism, emphasizing the need for caution when combining it with pharmaceuticals. These findings hold significant importance for the integration of pharmacology and natural therapies.

Research Supporting The Benefits Of Grape Seed Extract

Bagchi, D., et al. "Effects of Grape Seed Proanthocyanidin Extract on Oxidative Stress and Gene Expression Related to Apoptosis." Nutrition and Cancer (2002).

This study investigates the impact of grape seed proanthocyanidin extract (OPCs) on oxidative stress and its role in regulating genes associated with apoptosis, highlighting the potential protective role of grape seed in cancer prevention.

Kaur, M., et al. "Grape Seed Extract Inhibits Growth of Human Colorectal Cancer Cells In Vitro and In Vivo." Clinical Cancer Research (2006).

This research demonstrates that grape seed extract effectively inhibits the growth of human colorectal cancer cells both in vitro and in vivo, underscoring its potential as an adjunctive therapy in cancer treatment.

Agarwal, C., et al. "Anticancer Efficacy of Grape Seed Extract Against Human Breast Cancer Cells." Breast Cancer Research and

Treatment (2004).

This study reveals that grape seed extract suppresses the proliferation of human breast cancer cells, suggesting its promising application in breast cancer therapy.

Bagchi, D., et al. "Role of Grape Seed Extract Rich in Proanthocyanidins in Reducing Oxidative Stress and Inflammation in Chronic Diseases." Molecular Nutrition & Food Research (2008).

This study explores the ability of grape seed extract to reduce oxidative stress and inflammation associated with chronic diseases, emphasizing its potential benefits in preventing and managing various illnesses.

Tyagi, A., et al. "Grape Seed Extract Induces Apoptosis in Human Prostate Cancer Cells." Molecular Carcinogenesis (2003).

The research identifies that grape seed extract induces apoptosis in human prostate cancer cells, indicating its possible application in prostate cancer therapy.

Bagchi, D., et al. "Immunomodulatory Effects of Grape Seed Proanthocyanidin Extract in Cancer." Nutrition and Cancer (2003).

This study examines the immunomodulatory properties of grape seed extract, suggesting its supportive role in cancer treatment.

Background and Applications of Traditional

Chinese Medicine (TCM)

Foundations of TCM

Traditional Chinese Medicine is rooted in the interplay of complex philosophical principles that are increasingly supported by modern research and scientific evidence. Advances in pharmacology have expanded the applications of traditional herbal medicine, bridging ancient wisdom with modern medical practices.

China Academy Of Chinese Medical Sciences

http://www.catcm.ac.cn/

The China Academy of Chinese Medical Sciences is one of the most authoritative institutions in TCM research, specializing in scientific studies, education, healthcare, and international collaboration. The academy conducts extensive fundamental and clinical research on topics such as cancer treatment, immune regulation, and anti-aging. Its findings provide robust scientific support for the modernization of TCM and significantly advance the integration of traditional Chinese medicine with contemporary medicine.

Huangdi Neijing (The Inner Canon Of The Yellow Emperor)

The Huangdi Neijing is a cornerstone of traditional Chinese medicine, a timeless classic encompassing over 2,000 years of knowledge about life and health. It emphasizes the critical role of Qi, blood circulation, and the balance of Yin and Yang in maintaining well-being. By exploring the mysteries of the human body, this text deciphers the keys to health. According to its theories, the onset of diseases, including cancer, is closely linked to disruptions in Qi and blood flow, as well as imbalances in Yin and Yang. As such, TCM principles for cancer treatment focus on regulating Qi and blood and restoring Yin-Yang balance. Methods such as acupuncture, herbal medicine, and dietary adjustments aim to rebalance the body's internal environment, thereby preventing and treating diseases.

Shanghan Lun (Treatise On Cold Damage)

Written by the renowned Eastern Han physician Zhang Zhongjing, the Shanghan Lun is one of the most significant classics in TCM, primarily addressing externally contracted diseases, including infectious diseases. It systematically introduces the Six Channels Syndrome Differentiation theory and the principles of formula application, laying the foundation for syndrome differentiation and formula sciences in TCM. Even today, the Shanghan Lun serves as a critical reference in TCM clinical practice.

Shanghai University Of Traditional Chinese Medicine

http://www.shutcm.edu.cn/

As a leading institution in the field, the Shanghai University of Traditional Chinese Medicine excels in research on herbal medicine and cancer treatment. Extensive clinical and experimental studies conducted by the university provide scientific evidence supporting the effectiveness of herbal medicine in cancer recovery. For instance, certain traditional Chinese medicines have been shown to enhance the immune system, mitigate the side effects of chemotherapy and radiotherapy, and inhibit cancer cell growth. These findings offer valuable insights into integrating TCM into modern cancer therapies.

Accessing Related Literature and Research

Scholarly articles, papers, and research related to Huangdi Neijing and Shanghan Lun can be accessed through platforms such as China National Knowledge Infrastructure (CNKI) (https://www.cnki.net/) and the National Digital Library of China (https://www.nlc.cn/enweb/).

These four classics and institutions represent the core resources of TCM, encompassing theoretical foundations, clinical applications, pharmacological research, and modernization efforts. Together, they form the pillars of TCM's contributions to health management, particularly in cancer treatment.

Background and Authoritative Resources in Western Medicine

For detailed information on modern approaches to cancer treatment and insights into the causes of cancer, the following resources provide authoritative medical literature:

American Cancer Society (Acs)

https://www.cancer.org/

The American Cancer Society offers comprehensive information on cancer prevention, screening, and recovery, serving as a vital global source of cancer knowledge. Its resources include the latest research findings and lifestyle recommendations, empowering patients and their families to better manage the disease and improve their quality of life.

American Society Of Clinical Oncology (Asco)

https://www.asco.org/

ASCO provides extensive resources on the latest advancements in cancer treatment and research, supporting clinicians and researchers with up-to-date information. These resources contribute to improving the quality and innovation of cancer care globally.

National Cancer Institute (Nci)

https://www.cancer.gov/

The National Cancer Institute is a global leader in cancer research, providing authoritative insights into cancer biology, genetic factors, and treatment strategies. Through NCI, individuals can gain a deeper understanding of the complexities of cancer and the modern medical approaches used to combat it.

World Health Organization (Who)

https://www.who.int/health-topics/cancer

The World Health Organization delivers comprehensive reports on global cancer research and treatment, examining the role of environmental and genetic factors in cancer development. WHO's publications aim to foster international collaboration to enhance cancer prevention and treatment worldwide.

Integrating Western and Traditional Medicine

The literature and research summarized above offer valuable scientific support for integrating traditional Chinese medicine with modern oncology practices. By combining the wisdom of traditional medicine with advances in contemporary medicine, readers can gain a more holistic understanding of cancer recovery pathways and make informed health decisions grounded in scientific evidence.

Appendix: Disclaimer on Natural Therapies and Supplements

In this book, we introduce various natural therapies and supplements that have been used in the process of combating cancer to address health challenges. To prevent potential misunderstandings or misinterpretations, we issue the following disclaimer.

Disclaimer is as follows:

In Chapter 5 and related sections of this book, we share in detail several natural therapies and supplements that we personally used during the cancer recovery process and found to be beneficial. These include Salvestrol, liquid zinc, THC cannabis oil, Vitamin C, Vitamin D3, among others. These therapies played a significant role in the recovery journey for both myself and Yulia. By sharing these experiences, we hope to offer valuable insights and support to others facing similar challenges.

However, it is important to emphasize that while these supplements were helpful in our recovery, they represent personal experiences shared for informational purposes only. They are not intended as advertisements or universal recommendations.

As mentioned in the main text, a balanced diet typically provides adequate nutrition for healthy individuals. For those with specific health conditions or unique needs, it is crucial to consult a qualified healthcare professional before undertaking any health measures to ensure their safety and suitability.

Conclusion

This chapter aims to provide readers with supplementary information on natural therapies, relevant research resources, and authoritative references to serve as a broader foundation for support. When facing significant health challenges such as cancer, the integration of scientific research, personal experiences, and professional medical guidance is crucial. While every individual's recovery journey is unique, obtaining comprehensive information, cultivating a healthy lifestyle, and following professional advice can establish a solid foundation for recovery and longevity.

We hope that the insights and experiences shared in this book not only inspire each reader but also offer strength and support, empowering you to overcome life's challenges and embark on a healthier, more fulfilling path forward.

AFTERWORD

As you reach the final page of this book, we sincerely hope you have felt the power of faith and the warmth of support through these true stories. Each cancer warrior's resilience and determination not only highlight the greatness of the human spirit but also demonstrate how, even in the darkest moments, strength can be found through inner belief and the support of those around us. May these stories ignite hope within you and provide the courage to move forward.

The fight against cancer is not only a medical challenge but also a profound journey of the soul. This journey demands unwavering determination and relies heavily on the presence of family, friends, and professional teams. Every person who stands by your side, offering their support, is a vital source of strength to help you overcome obstacles. Please believe that while the path is filled with challenges, steadfast faith and a positive mindset are powerful tools in defeating illness.

We hope this book serves not just as a guide but also as a sanctuary for your heart. In the hustle and bustle of daily life, may you take moments to pause, focus on your health, and listen to your inner voice. On life's journey, may you lift your gaze to the future and cherish the beauty around you. No matter how arduous the road ahead may seem, light is always within reach.

Through this extraordinary journey of fighting cancer, may you find encouragement in these stories and remain steadfast in your belief in the power of health.

Let us walk this path together, bravely facing each new dawn filled with hope.

May health be a constant companion for you and your family, and may happiness always illuminate the road ahead in your life's journey.

ABOUT THE AUTHOR

Chunmei Yao

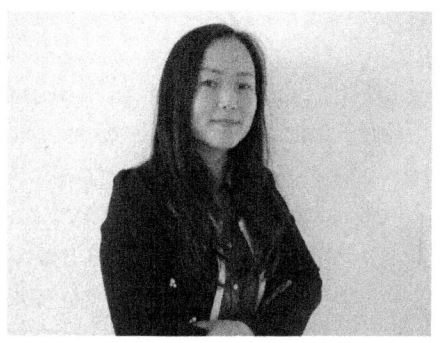

For many years, my work required me to shuttle frequently between Europe and Asia, with my annual flight mileage equating to six laps around the globe. The relentless time zone changes and high-intensity work rhythm left me chronically fatigued, depriving me of adequate rest. This high-pressure lifestyle gradually took a toll on my health and vitality, leaving visible marks on my well-being.

Through ongoing reflection, I came to realize that health is not a luxury or an afterthought but should be the foundation of life itself. As my introspection deepened, I began to understand that the essence of health is surprisingly simple and pure: almost anyone can achieve an ideal balance and a fulfilling life by maintaining a healthy weight, improving overall well-being, and preventing chronic illnesses. This does not require strenuous exercise or restrictive dieting but rather a balanced and sustainable lifestyle. This realization further reinforced my belief that so-called "obesity genes" are not a predetermined fate; with wise and proactive choices, anyone can find their unique path to health and balance.

From these profound insights, I compiled my learnings into two books: Restful Sleep Unlocked and The Art of Healthy Living. These books encapsulate my years of reflection and practice on health, specifically tailored for those who struggle with sleep quality and health management. I firmly believe that the content of these books will not only help you improve your overall state of well-being but will also have a lasting positive impact on your quality of life. Regardless of where you are in your journey, these simple and practical methods can guide you toward a path of better health.

In mid-2024, I had the privilege of engaging in a profound conversation with Mr. Leo Martin, a resilient cancer warrior who triumphantly overcame advanced cancer. As someone deeply passionate about health, I was profoundly moved by his extraordinary journey and those of other cancer survivors. Inspired, I felt a strong urge to document these stories in a book. When I proposed this idea, Leo generously agreed and selflessly shared every detail of his cancer battle, providing me with immense inspiration and support. His journey taught me about the resilience and miracles of life, leading to the creation of Overcoming and Healing Cancer: Inspiring True Stories of Recovery. This book reflects the profound insights drawn from this miraculous journey.

The book not only chronicles Leo Martin's extraordinary experience and his efforts to help others successfully combat cancer but also sheds light on how miracles of life can unfold in unexpected ways. It aims to provide hope and actionable strategies for those battling cancer or seeking to enhance their quality of life and improve their health. We hope that you will draw strength and confidence from its pages, face challenges with courage, and pursue harmony and recovery for both mind and body. May this book empower you to take control of your journey toward healing and renewal.

Finally, it is our heartfelt wish that this book inspires those in need of support during difficult times, offering an enduring courage to never give up. May each of us be a source of light, not only warming ourselves but also illuminating the path for others.

ACKNOWLEDGMENTS AND GRATITUDE

At the conclusion of this book, we extend our heartfelt gratitude to each courageous individual who selflessly shared their story. Your invaluable experiences in overcoming cancer have imparted wisdom and strength to every reader. It is through your unwavering support, love, and perseverance that I was able to collaborate with you to complete this book. Your honesty and bravery shine a light on the struggles and victories along the path of recovery, forming the very essence of this work. Your courage breathes life into these pages, making this book a cherished guide for countless individuals navigating their own journeys to healing.

I firmly believe that your experiences not only inspire those currently facing the trials of cancer but also offer hope and resilience to anyone in need of strength. By overcoming adversity, you have shown through your actions that even in moments of despair, hope and healing are still possible. For those walking a similar path, your stories serve as guiding lights, illuminating the way forward and helping them emerge from the darkness. May your bravery and resilience empower all who read this book, infusing new hope into the hearts of those still fighting.

We also express our profound respect to your families and friends. In the face of immense challenges, their steadfast support has been a source of strength, helping you overcome difficult times and reminding us that there is light at the end of the tunnel.

Special recognition is due to the medical professionals, researchers, and advocates dedicated to improving the lives of individuals affected by cancer. Your tireless efforts have reignited hope in countless lives, making a profound impact on many.

Additionally, I extend heartfelt thanks to Thomas for your extraordinary contributions to the successful completion of this book. From layout and design to every stage of publication, your dedication and meticulous attention to detail ensured that this book was presented in a visually appealing and accessible format, leading to its successful release.

Finally, to every reader who has taken the time to engage with this book, we offer our sincere appreciation. May you draw strength and inspiration from these pages and continue to share this love and courage with others who need it. Together, let us carry forward the messages of hope, healing, and resilience in the hearts of all.

Printed in Great Britain
by Amazon